Today's Stoic, Tomorrow's Hero?

Today's Stoic, Tomorrow's Hero?

Gerald T. Keep

iUniverse, Inc.

New York Lincoln Shanghai

Today's Stoic, Tomorrow's Hero?

iUniverse books may be ordered through booksellers or by contacting:

iUniverse
2021 Pine Lake Road, Suite 100
Lincoln, NE 68512
www.iuniverse.com
1-800-Authors (1-800-288-4677)

ISBN-13: 978-0-595-36814-3 (pbk)
ISBN-13: 978-0-595-67423-7 (cloth)
ISBN-13: 978-0-595-81228-8 (ebk)
ISBN-10: 0-595-36814-X (pbk)
ISBN-10: 0-595-67423-2 (cloth)
ISBN-10: 0-595-81228-7 (ebk)

Printed in the United States of America

Contents

   Facing up to mortality.
   Leaving a special memory behind.

   Sharing a dream.
   Common values, uncommon backgrounds.

   Forging a union.
   Family Traditions.
   The first seeds of disappointment.

   Adopting our children.
   Family problems of a mobile workforce.
   Sincerity in networking.
   Return to community.
   Building a Family.

   Solving the wrong problem.
   The early stages of liver disease.
   When disease undermines who you are.

Acknowledgements & Dedication

Acknowledgement

I'd like to thank the doctors, nurses, therapists, and counselors, all of whom did what they could for us.

I'd like to thank the incredibly extended community of people who helped me and my family get through these years, each in their own way.

Finally, I'd like to thank my readers, Dr. Tony Bower, Danielle Houser, Virginia Keep, and Linda Waltner, each of whom is very special in my life, each in their own way.

Dedication

This book is dedicated to all the survivors who struggle on stoically, to my boys, whose privacy I've tried to protect, and of course to Lynda, in hopes that something good will come from her suffering.

Foreword

A hero faces danger and hardship voluntarily to achieve some higher goal; stoics endure danger and hardship because they have no other choice short of the grave. Throughout the events I describe in this book, I have felt like a stoic, with no choice but to endure, while countless friends and even strangers have told me what inspiration they have drawn from our example. For me to turn away from supporting my family would have been to turn my back on everything I value in my life; perhaps heroes feel the same way, and it is the higher ideal that makes the difference. If you too can find inspiration from this chronicle, perhaps you can find the difference between a stoic and a hero.

1

Our Last Christmas?

	Winter	Spring	Summer	Fall
1996				(1) Christmas

It was late in the holiday season when Lynda figured that she was dying.

It had not been a good year for her. Her monthly cramps had gotten progressively more severe until a diagnosis of "endometriosis" put a name to the pain. This condition results from the escape of tissue normally lining the uterus out into the abdominal cavity, where it causes adhesions of a woman's sensitive organs to the abdominal wall. Responding to the normal menstrual cycles, it caused monthly episodes of unendurable agony that drove her to prescription pain killers, which were all the doctors could offer her. It eventually led to the total disintegration of her normal life.

Month by month the pains came and went, came and went, came—then stayed. Her abdomen swelled, and well meaning strangers would approach and ask when the baby was due—which was particularly hurtful to her since infertility had resulted in us having to adopt our children. The swelling made it uncomfortable to eat, and at our Thanksgiving gathering that year, friends and relatives tried hard not to notice that she ate very lightly. Most everyone assumed that she were dieting due to her apparent weight gain. By Christmas, a few mouthfuls of anything made her nauseous. Poor nutrition lead to anemia and fatigue. Something was wrong that mere painkillers could never cure.

Finally, Lynda was forced to overcome her fear of doctors and admit there might be a bigger problem, and so sought further help. Scans showed a large fluid-like mass in her abdomen. She might have cancer. More tests were required.

Faced with this, Lynda was sure this would be her last holiday and her boys would be left without a mother before the seasons marched around to another winter. She needed to *do* something. She fixated on the need to leave the boys with a special memory of something that we had done together as a family that they could treasure long after she was gone. Sure, we always had a Christmas tree and lit Hanukkah candles—anything we could recall from our own childhoods

1

with which to delight the children and forge a new set of family traditions. But Lynda wanted something more—something beyond just special.

Fortunately I had seen something in the holiday closing sales that sparked an idea. We bought an electric train and a set of village houses with wee lights, complete with little people, and a set of old-fashion globe street lights. We cleared off a big table in the library, spread a white sheet, and built a winter scene. As a finishing touch I sprinkled the whole lay-out with silver glitter. We turned out the room lights and enjoyed the sparkling fairy book village. We shivered together at the imaginary ice while the fireplace crackled in the next room and a cold breeze blew outside.

This was not the last time that our love for our children gave a purpose to our despair, nor was it the last time we assembled our winter village. Each year we would count the blessings that had gotten us through another year. Each year the village would grow as we added more buildings, fuzzy snow blanket, landscaping, roads, a skating pond. Each year we'd wonder whether we would have another full year together.

It turned out that Lynda's problem was not cancer but rather liver disease. The cause was never determined, though they ran her through every test in the book. I believe that the pain pills she took for the endometriosis resulted in enough liver damage and scarring to push her over the line into crisis. We'll never know for sure.

What we did learn was that a person's entire blood supply moves through a person's liver, and that hers was no longer up to the demands placed on it. To force the issue, the Portal vein that feeds the liver had developed a huge back-pressure (called Portal Hypertension). This forced the blood through the liver but also caused leakage of fluid from the veins. This leaking fluid pooled up in her abdomen, causing the swelling that led to the other events, one linked to another in a chain.

The short-term treatment was fluid control ranging from limiting salt intake, to diuretics, to physically draining the excess fluids with needles.

The long-term treatment was a liver transplant—if a compatible liver could be found. Usually this meant someone would have to die and no longer need theirs. The waiting list was long, and there was no way of knowing how sick Lynda would get, or how fast.

Only time would tell.

2

Courtship

	Winter	Spring	Summer	Fall
1988	(2) Engagement			
1996				(1) Christmas

Lynda and I met in 1987, about a year after we had both followed our careers to Appalachia. Our mutual interest was international folk dance, and we met on the wooden floor of the University gymnasium. At this time most of the group was married couples; there were few singles. Lynda was just ending a long-term relationship with an old boy friend. I was just settling into my new career in industry and looking around for that right someone with whom to start a family.

Many people recommend church as a social environment suitable to seeking a spouse. Unfortunately for me, this region was far more fundamentalist than I was used to. It was traditional for women here to marry young—right out of high school. It did not feel right to go to a church which I would not have chosen otherwise, in search of female companionship.

But more to the point, I was seeking a strong woman who shared my values and would be a partner in life, not some young girl I would dominate by virtue of superior age, education, employability, or whatever. I wanted someone I could respect and look up to—someone I could count on to be strong and reliable, seasoned by passing through the fire; someone whom I could admire for who they were and what they had accomplished. And, someone flexible enough to put up with my own eccentricities, and who knew their own mind, but still chose in the end to be with me.

I found the kind of partner I *was* looking for in Lynda. She was a rather moderate Jew; I thought of myself as a Unitarian by upbringing, and had studied world religions in college, among other electives. We both came from backgrounds with a strong belief in love, tolerance, equal rights for all humankind regardless of race or gender—the kind of thing taught by Jesus but ignored in practice by so many who called themselves "Christians".

Her work was in early childhood development and special education, with a focus on birth to 3 year olds. She visited neonatal intensive care units (NICU's)

3

and followed preemies and sick newborns to learn how they would develop and what their special needs were. She helped screen babies from up in the coal country. Many of them were poor—in both money and education. But Lynda's eyes would sparkle as she described the big burly coal miners who came in carrying these tiny preemies that would almost fit in the palm of their hand (the ones that really could fit in the palm of a hand were in isolation units in the NICU). These people were ever so gentle and loving, but they just didn't know what to do for these specially challenged babies.

Lynda was on a 12-month contract at the University, writing more grants than teaching. Over her career she has pulled in over 70 million dollars of grant money (unheard of in an Education Department) to set up programs in the area for birth to 3 year olds with special needs.

She tells of a foster family with a baby that had severe handicaps that she helped keep alive, even getting in the oxygen tent with her and getting her to eat when no one else could. She helped this foster family learn to cope with the baby's debilitating handicaps. This developed into a long-term friendship, with Lynda helping in other ways with many other foster children passing through that family. They ultimately adopted many of those unfortunate children permanently. This friendship would bear unexpected fruit in Lynda's own time of need.

Here was a lady that loved children, but had none of her own. She was strong, and knew how to care for children. She was past her bloom of youth (how far past I was never completely sure till I saw it on the marriage license). She was soured on the prospects of marriage after a brief marriage to a fundamentalist Jewish man and other unsuccessful attempts at establishing a positive relationship with men since then. She was helping far more children in her career than she could raise in a single household and would find it very hard to justify sacrificing the good of the many by leaving her career for the good of a few, albeit her own.

What she lacked in youthful energy, I figured, I could make up for given my own interest in children and not inconsiderable housekeeping skills. I'm actually quite a "nester", who like to tinker and fix things around the house.

I'm a passable cook, especially baking. My mom started a tradition of elaborate birthday cakes, and I kept that up with the boys. I would recreate space ships, Lazer Tag battles, castle sieges, underwater scenes, and so forth. And not just for the boys—I made Lynda one memorable Dalmatian puppy cake on an early trip to the beach. The humidity was so high, the cake kept wanting to droop and the head fall off between the paws. It ended up having so many toothpicks in it to hold it together that it was almost dangerous to eat.

Simplistically I took on faith that our double income would fill the holes left in our ability to do all the chores traditionally assigned to each gender. I suppose in many ways it did. As much as it went against my middle-class grain we hired people to mow lawns, help clean, paint, and do jobs we both knew how to do but hadn't the time for.

She had reached an age where she was unlikely to have children—with no other prospects in sight. Her biological clock was winding down. I recognized that I had a chance to dramatically leverage her contribution to the next generation. By choosing to partner up with someone like Lynda who would not otherwise have had kids, I would be increasing the number of Good People who are engaged in raising our next generation. I could give her the gift of motherhood and help her raise a family the best way I knew, with two active and involved parents. I had a happy childhood and a good model of parenting. Lynda had an unhappy childhood and strong ideas of what she would do differently.

What about love? I was old enough to know the difference between love and lust (and yes, there was enough of that to hold our interest—we were both particularly fond of massages). The temporary fringe benefit of having a pretty, young wife in bed at night was far less important to me than having a woman of proven character, steel tempered "by passing through the fire". Those strengths are characteristics that would last a lifetime and could be counted on (of course I had no idea what I'd be learning about how fragile the human conscious mind can be).

I stayed in school until I was 25, earning a PhD both because it was easy for me and because I had faith that more education meant better financial support of that hoped-for family when the time came. By whatever grace, I avoided the common pitfall of an early termination of my studies by an unplanned conception.

For me I saw the strength of family upbringing and the failure of absentee fathers as a major crying need in our society. And of course graduating with a PhD put me far enough ahead on a career path (and that esthetic scale of scientific contribution to the knowledge of mankind) that I felt I had some slack to give there. What was missing for me by staying in school so long and moving to a distant region for a job, was family.

All in all, partnering with Lynda seemed the best choice I could make. We had many mutual interests and enjoyed each other's company. There was enough sexual attraction to keep things interesting. As I learned that a 12-year gap separated us, I was not swayed in my resolve. I felt my extreme IQ (pointed out repeatedly in my youth by parents who cared about my achievements as well as my happiness) in some way counterbalanced some of her experience advantage, putting us on more even footing. She was obviously no dummy herself, having earned a PhD. In addition she had very rich experiences behind her that made me look like a wall flower.

She assured me that her age would not prevent her from having children, and as far as I was concerned she was the expert in such things. She knew much of modern medicine and much older people than she were having first children these days. She knew the risks to mother and child, and I couldn't think of anyone in a better position to know, given her work.

She was really more concerned with the other end of our prospective children's childhood. She did not want to be retiring before the kids left college, so her window of opportunity was there, but was fleeting.

I still do not fault my reasons or my choices. Later, as things fell apart, I was tempted to consider how much of a factor Lynda's age was in all her eventual difficulties. My values and my thinking about what is important in life preparative to making this choice served me well as I navigated the rocks in our future. Our mutual commitment to do right by the children was a powerful beacon that could cut through any fog and take the measure of any problem.

3

Our Wedding

	Winter	Spring	Summer	Fall
1988	(2) Engagement	**(3) Wedding**		
1996				(1) Christmas

It was at a dinner concert in 1987, with wonderful Madrigal singers whom we enjoyed immensely, that I asked Lynda to come home with me that Christmas and meet my parents, for mutual introductions and to show off both ways—parents and fiancée—as I was very proud of both.

On her part, she assured me she would not expect me to have to deal with her own parents, with whom she had a strong love-hate relationship going. Indeed she vowed she would do her best to shelter me from them, such were her feelings at that time. For all that, she spoke with her mother on the phone more than I did with my own, with whom I got along marvelously. I was aggressively civilized when we met, so was able to hold my own.

We agreed to raise our children in an open religious environment as Unitarians—each of us bringing into the family whatever traditions we treasured from our own childhoods. We would celebrate Christmas *and* Passover, hunt Easter eggs *and* spin the dreidel at Hanukkah. It was only through Lynda that I learned the fun holiday games you play with gold foil covered chocolate coins. I taught her the joy of Ukrainian Easter Egg dying, with wax applications to protect parts of a painting as it went through stages of darker and darker colored dyes.

As a kid at Christmas, we did a lot of special things in my family. We would make a dozen different kinds of cookies and have a big frosting party—I actually kept this up in graduate school to the amusement of my friends, and of course involved the boys as soon as they could hold a spoon. We'd decorate a tree and put up lights—and only fight a little over the tastefulness of white-only lights vs. splurging in glorious flashing colors. We'd write letters to Santa Claus, and left a piece of red felt in the fireplace screen, telling the boys that Santa had caught his pants on the way out. We left milk and cookies for Santa and a carrot for Rudolf (all of which were half-eaten by morning). I wanted all this for my boys.

We both thought some formal religious exposure was important to raising kids and the Unitarians were the best choice for us in the area. So it was natural for us to seek out a Unitarian minister for our wedding the next spring. We described our plans—modeled after what we had heard of a Quaker service, in which you sit in a circle with all your fiends and family, with quiet time for reflection, and each person standing to share their thoughts or give an offering of music, until at the end the couple rose and exchanged vows.

The minister we needed to make it all legal was in the process of leaving the community. She expressed her discomfort with taking on the role we described and declined the honor. On reflection, we realized there really was no place for a minister neither of us knew in the ceremony that we wanted; we were exchanging our vows as responsible adults in front of friends and family—all the people we cared about in the world that we could gather.

In the end we recognized the needs of law and of community were quite independent. In fact we went to a Justice of the Peace for a marriage license the day before the *real* ceremony. We took only two local mutual friends as witnesses and downplayed the importance of that part.

We called for the gathering to be Memorial Day Weekend 1988 as friends and family flocked in from all over the country. In some ways it was like a family reunion. We had a pot-luck reception after a lovely ceremony in our large backyard (which, ironically, several guests later pointed out was decorated with poison ivy).

Thus I have a unique excuse for not "remembering" our anniversary. We signed the license on the 27th and had the public ceremony Sunday the 28th, but really it was all pegged to Memorial Day Weekend, so our anniversary float over several possible days depending on when the last Monday in May falls, and how you choose to figure it.

The ceremony was exactly what we hoped for. We easily had over a hundred with us that day, and musical offerings ranged from recorder and flute to hammer dulcimer. At one point I rose and described the wedding rings that we had had custom made in rose and white gold. There is a rope braid along each edge with three symbols along the band. Mine is inside round with a taper for comfort while hers is more cylindrical since she was more used to wearing rings. The central symbol is a maple leaf to symbolize childhood—we both grew up in wet eastern climates with maple tress before moving west to drier climates later in life. The two symbols flanking are our favorite flowers (my choice a rose, hers a daisy) symbolizing each of our ideals that would be joined to create again a new generation's childhood, a new family.

We were going to flank these symbols by a pair of pine cones, the symbology of which we didn't delve into too deeply (following the western adult life-line motif I guess) when the goldsmith pointed out that the bumps at that point on the ring would cut into adjacent fingers and be quite uncomfortable—so we left them out. Hence the pine cones came to symbolize the trials and tribulations in adult life which we hoped to leave out of our futures as well.

Lynda did not want a diamond engagement ring. Her first diamond was hocked to pay the mortgage after her first marriage went sour, and she saw it as a wasteful vanity for a couple just starting out. It also symbolized a dowry and "buying" the bride, chauvinistic sentiments we both found distasteful, so I went with her wishes. She spoke of maybe wanting a diamond on our tenth anniversary, when we could far better afford a very nice one.

Before the wedding, Lynda was so keyed up and on cloud nine that she couldn't focus on getting ready. Her childhood friend, the sister she almost had, at whose house she spent more time as a kid than at her own, was with her in the bedroom, trying to get her ready. Lynda would drift off on some tangent down memory lane, and her "sister" would say "that's nice Lynda, now put on your dress."

As everyone waited outside, the helium balloons decorating the yard began to warm up in the sun and started to go off—punctuating the happy sounds of the gathering. Everyone joked about it being a shot-gun wedding of a very different sort!

Lynda eventually joined us, and the ceremony went off well, punctuated by the occasional balloon also going off.

We had agreed on vows to exchange—not about honor and obey until "death do us part" but rather about love, support, and encouraging mutual growth. I'm sure I got the words right though I can't remember them exactly now; we've got it on tape thanks to friends. Lynda was so flustered, happy, and overcome by the whole scene that all she could say was, basically, "Me too!"

There followed quite a party in which Lynda revealed to all that she had persuaded me to wear tiger-stripped bikini briefs under my formal gray suit—by promising not to tell—and a good time was had by all.

We abandoned the house to the much-extended family, and retired to a room at a hotel a friend of ours managed. There Lynda took a second shot at remembering her vows in the Jacuzzi tub. She didn't find all the words we'd agreed on, but she hit all the high points.

As the tension of this highly emotional day drained out of her there in the hot luxurious tub, one point of tension did not fade, but instead got worse. Something was hurting her inside, bad.

So, instead of exploring her anatomy the way I had expected to on our wedding night, we proceeded to the emergency room to examine her anatomy with ultrasound imaging. This disclosed a benign fibroid tumor in her uterine wall. Since this was all the doctors found, we were left to assume that it had somehow flared up due to all the excitement—though how or why that worked no one could explain to us. Things got better with pain killers and sedatives, and we were able to return to the house the next morning and pretend it had never happened. An odd blot it was on an otherwise wonderful wedding weekend, which was in fact a dark foreshadowing of things to come.

4

Finding Help

	Winter	Spring	Summer	Fall
1988	(2) Engagement	(3) Wedding		
89-95	**(4) Raising our Children**			
1996				(1) Christmas

In one sense, we needed help raising a family from the very beginning; for reasons I'll go into later, we couldn't have biological children. So, we chose to go the adoption route.

The ironic thing about adopting was that, from conception to arrival, it took the same nine months to do the paperwork as it would have taken to carry a baby to term. And, from the man's perspective at least, it was at least as painful.

Lynda, with her Early Childhood Education background, was well placed to investigate the different programs available for placing children in need of a family. This also meant that she was aware of how critical the early months, and even prenatal care, were to the baby's neuro-physical development. Thus she did not want to get an older child with problems, or one that had gone through foster care. She wanted as close to a newborn as possible. She was also advised that many of the troubled young women in our area that were offering their future babies up for adoption at birth, were either suffering from mental health problems, or had alcohol or drug habits, which can have devastating effects on a baby. We were drawn towards overseas programs where children were in need due to poverty, but less likely to be from mothers who were dealing with substance abuse.

Each adoption program catered to a different clientele. Many of the programs were funded by a particular religious group, and were only available to members of their specific faith. With our patch-work religious background, many of these were not open to us. Others had an age restriction and Lynda had just turned forty, so those were out. There were no programs yet coming out of Eastern Europe at that time. Many children were coming out of China, but generally these were at least a year old, because they had spent time in an orphanage and now were old enough to be flown to the US by an agency. Lynda wanted a newborn, to bond with and nurture properly, so our best hope was Central or South America.

United States emigration law was such that adoption and entry into the country was easiest if the mother was available to waive her rights and testify that the father was unknown. The laws of each country of origin, however, were different one to the next. It was theoretically possible to adopt a child under some country's laws, then be unable to bring that child back into the States. We did not want to plow new ground here; one must stick with an established program. Some programs had as much as an eight month waiting period, whereby the adoptive parents basically had to come, start the process, then go back to the US and leave the child in someone else's care for that critical early period.

The best program for us turned out to be Peru. There was a civil war going on, with the Maoist Shining Path Guerrillas running a reign of terror in the country-side, killing the elected officials and any opposition. Many poor refugees were flocking to the cities. Under these conditions, many children needed homes and the system was geared to move fast. The adoptive parents would take custody immediately and at least one was expected to stay with the baby until the legal work was done—potentially as little as six weeks.

So, we began the process for adoption from Peru. We linked up with a local agency to do the home studies and began a series of investigations more intrusive than any a US employer would be allowed to conduct—certainly more than we do in selecting our political leadership. We had medical exams to be sure we were expected to live through raising the children, psychological exams to be sure we'd not abuse them, and financial investigations to be sure we could afford to raise them. We had background checks run through the local police, the FBI, and even Interpol. I gained a disturbing insight into forensic investigation that I might never have gotten otherwise, when they had to try several times, even under perfect conditions, back and forth, to get a set of my fingerprints that the agencies considered readable. Only Sherlock Holmes could deduce a criminal's biography from the simple inky smudges law officers actually have to go on.

Every document had to be notarized. Then these documents had to be certified at the county level, showing that this was the seal of a bona fide notary. The State then had to certify that the county certification was valid, following which the entire collection of documents was sent to the Peruvian embassy in Washington, DC. to be certified that these were all in proper order—for a fee of course. This was just a taste of the things to come.

Finally, we were ready to go. We were actually given a choice between a newborn boy and a six month old girl. While I really wanted a girl, Lynda's concerns carried the day.

Fees and expenses to be paid to the Peruvian lawyer were $7,000. We investigated secure wire transfers and all had about a 30% surcharge, so we decided to carry cash. I went into the bank and asked for seven $1,000 bills and was informed that such were no longer circulated. I had to take seventy $100 bills. A stack of seventy bills is about a half inch thick—too big to put in a wallet, and bigger than any money belt we could find. Eventually they were wrapped in a bundle and rode to Peru secured around my neck by a shoestring.

There was a hotel called Suite Service that catered to adoptive families there in Peru. We made our reservations, and arranged to be met at the airport by the hotel's car. Having done everything we could think of, we crossed our fingers and boarded the airplane.

They weren't fooling about taking custody of the baby immediately; we arrived Wednesday, took custody Thursday, and then our luggage arrived Friday. Thank goodness for all the other adoptive families at Suite Service—they were able to let us have extra baby gear until our carefully packed treasure trove of baby clothes, bottles, and above all, disposable diapers arrived.

At the lawyer's office we received the 4-week old baby directly from the arms of his birth mother. She was a 24-year old university student who was becoming involved with a man who didn't want to raise another man's son. Where many of the native Indian stock were short, typically under 5 feet due to a mixture of genetics and poor diet, she was from a prosperous farm in the country and was nearly as tall as I was.

The baby was darling. Even at that young age he tried to engage every eye in the room and smiled if you looked at him. He was going to be a people person. His big dark eyes were only exceeded in size by the lawyer's when I pulled the cash out from under my shirt. He wrote us out an artistic receipt and signed it with a grand masterpiece of a signature almost suitable for framing. We were hurried back to Suite Service and that was the last time we had to hurry during our entire stay.

The families at Suite Service banded together, waiting each day to see whether the lawyer's helpers would come and guessing who might have appointments with what government official that day. I don't think I ever saw the lawyer again—all the work was done by several young ladies in his employ who spoke excellent English—far, far better than his, at any rate.

We families were all in this together, with the veterans teaching the newer ones the ropes. This was our best source of information about the legal system, about the practical aspects of how to take care of babies, and about where to go to buy things. Most important, we learned where to go for pediatric medical attention, and what parts of town to avoid.   .

The Peruvian economy was in free fall. A friend later gave us a little gold coin smaller than a dime, called a "sol", Spanish for "sun". On a gold standard that might be worth about $60 but the "sol" had been devalued 1,000 sols to an "inti" and when we arrived there were 5,000 inti's to the dollar. They would put nine 1,000-inti bills together and staple a tenth around their middle to simplify counting. So at face value this $60 gold coin was worth less than a "green stamp"—a fraction of a fraction of a penny. When I left two and a half weeks later, the exchange rate was about 8,000 to a dollar. When Lynda left after eight and a half weeks, it was over 15,000 to the dollar. The fishing fleet was being devastated because the government mandated that half of all profits be put in the bank to save for new boats—but in intis so that it was quickly worth nothing. Nearly every street corner in Lima had a man with an electronic calculator who claimed to know the current exchange rate and would give you intis for dollars. We were directed to a local church where they gave an honest rate, converting their weekly collection plate into dollars for safety.

Everywhere I went, with my red gringo beard, it seemed I encountered a little girl in the street trying to sell me a pretty rock, or a little boy offering to polish my tennis shoes for me. I quickly developed a siege mentality and a gruff manner to protect myself emotionally from the poverty. Money meant so much more to them than to us, but if we were not firm we would drown in begging children and not be able to turn around. We tried to pay generously for the abundant craft work—some of it quite good—but inevitably held back funds out of caution. We had no idea how long we would be there, or what it would cost, or how we could get more cash from the States. Afterwards, we all wished we had bought more. Restaurant prices were about half of similar fare in the US—but the cost was almost entirely the raw materials—service cost almost nothing.

The only other sign of unrest was the fact that every nice house had a wall around it and every really important building, public or private, had a man standing out front with a machine gun. It was quite dangerous—for the guard, actually. The guerrillas were known to kill such people in order to get their guns.

The adopting families, mostly American, would go on outings together. It was quite a sight seeing a troop of Americans with strollers and diaper bags winding their way through a marketplace. Lynda, with her Mediterranean features and black hair, did not stand out like the rest of us, especially so since we used a "snuggly sack"—a sort of sling arrangement for the baby to ride on your front—rather than a stroller. One time Lynda sat down on the bench and a local woman sat down next to her, pointed at the caravan of baby strollers and said, "Look! See there? Those are Americans. They've come here to adopt all those babies." Lynda was constantly surprised at how strangers would come up to her and start giving advice on how to care for a newborn—how to dress them, how to feed them, and so forth.

A favorite outing was to the "Liverpool" restaurant. It was painted up with silhouettes of the Beatles. There you could get the best hamburger and pizza in Lima. If you were really, really brave you could try a salad since they made a point of washing everything in bottled water. Of course the bacteria in the local water were not compatible with what we carried with us in our own GI tracks. Eventually, everybody let something slip past their guard—ice cubes from local water in their drink, a garnish of onions washed in local water, something. The result was one extremely violent purging in the middle of the night, and then we were fine. Everybody did it once.

The exciting trip everybody went on was a trip to a ruined Inca city near Lima that was just beginning to be excavated. Many pyramids and such still lay beneath centuries of dirt.

We loaded up in a half-dozen of the ubiquitous VW bugs (made in Brazil) that served as taxis. The guide spent a moment worrying about my wire-frame glasses. We would be driving through some rough sections of the suburbs and he worried that someone might think the frames were real gold and try to steal them.

Traffic in Lima is fascinating. There are lines painted on the well engineered and paved city thoroughfares, but the lines are ignored. On 3-lane highways with street-lights, about five VW's can crowd up in the front row of cars. Few had seat-belts and none had working a/c so we rode with the windows open.

The poor section of town was less well paved, and looked like the dry desert that was natural to the area. Most of the people in the street were poorer Indians rather than more urban dressed Castilians. We stopped at one corner and a guy reached in the window and ripped the watch right off my wrist, breaking the band. All the ladies were horrified because I was holding the baby and the man could have hurt him—but clearly the whole incident was driven by poverty—I didn't begrudge him the watch. The tour guide was mortified and insisted on waiving the cost of my tour, saying it was his fault—he should have had us roll up the windows (in that heat!)

The ruins were fascinating. I found the guides ironic as they kept referring to the FEE-lion motifs in the stones. Then they encouraged tipping

I began to worry about the lack of shade for the baby and found myself seeking out every cool shadow beneath an old stone wall I could find. The baby insisted on turning his head a certain way in the snuggly sack and by time we got back to the Suites, the left half of his face was mildly sunburned. It was striking how the transition from red to tan split right down the middle of his nose, and made him look somewhat clownish. He looked painted. Lynda worried terribly about having to go in front of the Judge soon, them taking one look at the baby and accusing us of child abuse. But nothing moved that fast in Peru and a few days passed waiting for the next court appointment, and so too did the burn. It was rather sobering that about 10 days later, two lady officials spent about 5 minutes discussing what shade of skin tone they should put down for the baby in the legal court records.

After two and a half weeks, everything was in process and I headed home, leaving Lynda and the baby in company of Lynda's old college chum "Auntie", who had been able to join us there.

The wait back home seemed unnecessarily long, as each official in the chain demanded their due before they would sign. The judiciary branch of the government was trying to crack down on graft, corruption, and bribery. At one point, the judge had accused the Chief of Police of taking bribes and he was insulted enough to refuse to sign any more papers—shutting us down for awhile. It was said that he was trying to buy his daughter a piano. Eventually our lawyer figured out what the standard "gratuity" was and the wheels began to turn again. Yes, we had to bribe the chief law enforcement officer of the capital city in order to be allowed to provide a home for their unwanted children.

These kids of course had no idea how lucky they were. It takes a family of some means to travel to Peru. One little boy, 7 years old, was found living in a cardboard box in the streets and was so happy now to be joining a family with both a mother and a father. He informed them with glee that he knew a recipe for strawberry jam and that he and his mother could stay home together to make jam while the father went out to sell the jam on the street corners. In his mind, this meant that everything was going to be all right now. That was Roberto. His parents were probably killed by guerrillas. I can't imagine his reaction to arriving at their California estate, complete with swimming pool and every luxury. Roberto symbolized Peru for me. I often thought that at the very least, we had managed to save one little boy from Roberto's predicament. There would be one fewer boy trying to scrabble a meager living in the streets of Lima.

As the weeks wore on, the end came in sight. I got a call from Lynda saying that she thought she would be done by a certain date and that there was a flight through Panama City she thought she could catch. I was forced to inform her that she would <u>not</u> be on that flight, that the US had just invaded Panama and that Peru had broken off diplomatic relations with the US in protest.

But finally the papers were all signed and Lynda and the baby made it home on Christmas Eve, 1989.

Our second adoption was much less of an adventure. The agency doing our home monitoring following our adoption knew that we wanted another child. One day they called and said there was a biracial baby about to be born in the city that was being offered up by the mother for adoption at birth—would we like him? What could we do but say yes? Piece of cake.

Raising children in a region where neither of us had family, while both of us had careers, could at times be quite a daunting task.

With Lynda's connections she sought out the best of childcare arrangements, but those were only good when the children were well. Whenever one ran a fever or tossed their cookies, we whipped out our Day timers to figure out which of us had more urgent meetings that we simply could not miss, and which of us stayed with the sick child. My employer was understanding to a point; often I would take the child duty during the day, head back to work when everyone else was leaving, pump up on Mountain Dew and see whether I could make it 'till dawn—especially if I could sleep in on a following Saturday. What a way to spend Friday night!

But this sort of thing was making us old fast, and it was clear we needed help of the kind that money wouldn't buy. How then could we set about finding a substitute for the family that we didn't have, when we discovered that we really needed it?

We are not the first couple to discover this problem. Modern material wealth depends on having a cadre of highly trained technical experts to run things—a college educated upper middle class. But, to fulfill their role in society, these people must go where the jobs are, and where their particular skills are in demand, leaving behind family and friends, even those they had just grown close to in the formative years of college.

Thus in trying to serve society (granted they may not think of it that way at the time), they often separate themselves from it. Cast on new soil, how to find new roots?

In today's high-pressure media world, there are hundreds of smiling faces we see every day offering to be our "friend" for their own commercial or political reasons. We learn to mistrust the smiling faces with shallow hidden motives. We consider them phony low-lifes, and shudder at the thought of being in any way like them.

How then do we re-integrate ourselves into society without feeling like mercenaries? I've known many childish people who dealt with their "friends" on a quid-pro-quo basis. "I was nice to *them* so they *have* to be nice to me," or, "They owe me a birthday present." Others show tremendous outbursts of negative feelings over a forgotten birthday, anniversary, or holiday. Indeed I often feel such debts, and it takes the joy out of giving.

But if I despise the salesman, the mercenary, the greedy ones, how can I try to fit myself into a social network with full knowledge and desire to benefit from it without feeling like a hypocrite?

The answer is to exclude personal debt from the equation. Pay forward, not back. If you help someone and they express gratitude, tell them you know that they will help someone else in turn. Do not look for a pay-back, or worry too much about paying back those who have helped you. Look for ways to help when and where you can help best.

Do this and you become part of a community of caring and giving people. People will know you for who you are and will be grateful for opportunities they find to help you, when you make your needs known. They too can find joy in helping where there is no mercenary expectation, no counting of personal debt. An opportunity to help is an opportunity to "earn" the benefits and good will that one has already received gratis, and to feel more legitimately part of the community.

Cultivate friends and help them all in the ways that you, as a unique individual, can. Each of them will help someone, somewhere, and the world will be enriched. By being a contributing part of that, someone, somewhere, may find that they are able to help you when you most need it—perhaps in ways you could not imagine, let alone ask for.

This is about a life choice. You are not entering a business deal, or even a marriage. You are not "buying" friendship; you are choosing to be part of a team, a contributing member of society. It is not unlike choosing a political party or a religion.

"What goes around, comes around," they say. If you have faith in society, in community, and commit yourself to serving it, being part of it—you will find that you are not alone, and have more friends than you know. The transition from an individual-property mind-set to true community involvement is the achievement of a level of maturity that comes hard to those like me who have achieved personal wealth (some, anyway) and status (we'd like to think) through individual effort in our educational system—we of the educated upper middle class who have torn ourselves up by the roots. The people most in need of community hold the worst mental attitudes for achieving it. If one recognizes this, and manages to achieve the shift in values or perspective needed—not a phony sell-out, but actually develops a genuine desire to help and be involved in a broader community—then life becomes more enjoyable and much more worth living.

Lynda and I, two uprooted PhD's (and Damn Yankees to boot) came to Appalachia. We both tried to serve—Lynda through her work with children, I through involvement with Big Brothers, Church, Scouts, Soccer, and employment that may not have much direct social value but allowed me to contribute a couple dozen jobs to the community.

Soccer was great fun with the boys. Our oldest was very tentative about joining up and trying out, but once he was on a team, he really took to the group socialization and teamwork. Our youngest enjoyed the sport in the purest form, a natural athlete and show-off, when he wasn't chasing butterflies or wrestling on the side lines with the other kids. I ended up coaching his team for a few years. Watching my boys develop and grow was a real kick—you can see it so clearly in a focused arena like that. But of course I was aware that I was helping to develop other peoples' children as well, and greatly enjoyed rising to the responsibility, encouraging and supporting them.

Leading cub scouts was a great joy too. My youngest didn't like it—too much sharing and taking turns—but my oldest gloried in it. I got the kids building marble race tracks and newspaper bridges as team competitions. Once I let them pull the guts out of an old ruined VCR and they went absolutely berserk, like a shark feeding frenzy. They had never done such a thing before. Scavenger hunts and our first camping. A wonderful time. I was proud that of the dozen that started in that age group, I was able to keep six interested enough to move on to Boy Scouts.

Yes, we helped many people, but when our time of gravest need came, our story spread to hundreds we had never even met. Strangers would approach me, telling me that Lynda was on their church's prayer list, and offering to help in any way they could. This is not pay-back for the things we did. Our story spread because we were connected to the community. We were really connected to these "strangers" by a network of people, each link formed lovingly by the selfless giving of its members to their nearest neighbor.

The warm glow of belonging that we received could never come from quid-pro-quo relationships. The surprising magnitude of the response perhaps comes from being such a visible example of what community is all about. How could we ever pay that back? Not possible. But if our story in any way can help you, I will happily consider it a measure of paying forward.

Lynda and I had eight good years to build a family before the swelling in her abdomen put us into crisis.

Our first boy "came home" on Christmas Eve and I put up my first Christmas tree as a head of household, in anticipation of their arrival. My small 3-bedroom home that I had bought as a bachelor seemed perfect for a family of three. Lynda had sewed baby quilts with nursery rhyme shapes and we had prepared a nursery with paint and TLC.

Our eldest son was very people-oriented from the beginning. As a baby he would try to catch the eye of anyone in the room and when they looked, he smiled a big grin. He was always very careful and cautious. Crawling, if he bonked his head it was an absolute disaster and he'd cry, not because he was hurt but because of his sense of failure. Shortly after he learned to walk, I caught him pacing slowly across the living room one foot carefully placed ahead of the other. When he got to the end, he then started walking *backwards*, one foot behind the other just as carefully. The little bugger was *practicing* walking!

We took him to "Christmas in the Smokies" at Dollywood. He loved the lights that made every tree and bush seem magical. He had so much fun on the kiddie rides that we couldn't get him to leave even as it got dark and cold. We eventually had to pry his frozen blue fingers off the controls of his little airplane to take him home. In hindsight, maybe that's why he loved taking trips to the airport. When one of us had to travel, he loved to watch the airplanes take off and land.

Our younger son was the opposite in may ways when he came along. He never bothered to crawl, it seemed, and he went straight to running when his legs were strong enough. He didn't care about crashes, and usually got the best of his older brother in any tussle because of his higher threshold for pain. He never went through an awkward coltish growth spurt and was one of the most naturally coordinated and athletically gifted kids I've ever seen. On the other hand, his reaction to every new person who tried to hold him was to squirm, poke an elbow in their ribs, and throw up on them. He had no patience for watching airplanes and it turned out he was ADHD. Later he developed bipolar problems. One wonders about pre-natal effects. In nursery school, he would climb shelves to steal coffee from the teachers and they couldn't figured out why their mugs were mysteriously emptier for the longest time. Fortunately, with Lynda's connections, we had him diagnosed and on some stabilizing medication before kindergarten.

With two bundles of boy energy in my small bachelor's house, it was time to find something larger. We stretched our budget and went for a bigger house in the country.

Our first winter drove home to us what it meant to live on a hill when it snowed; the van simply couldn't make it up. So, half way up the icy hill, I stopped and let Lynda out with the boys while I took the van back down the hill to find a safe place to leave it.

Lynda told the eldest, who was three, to wait there for Daddy as she carried the baby up the treacherous track to the house. As I started back up the hill on foot, I heard a terrible wailing sound. I ran up the edge of the plowed road and saw where the little footprints followed along the road behind Mommy, right to the point where a boy could see our house through the trees. There, the footprints cut cross country. I followed them to find where he had fallen into a snow drift up to his armpits, but no worse for the wear. He was more frustrated than hurt. This is the boy who would grow up to be an avid camper with the Boy Scouts and brag about camping out in snow and worse. Go figure—is there a connection? They say what doesn't kill you makes you stronger.

The new house had a big carpeted play room where we could play at wrestling (the boys got a great thrill out of "pinning" Daddy). We started keeping tropical fish, many of which died from "ammonia" levels until I got the tanks balanced right. We would set up hundreds of dominos to fall in a row and had room to set up electric race tracks and leave them for a month at a time. We made massive landscapes out of Legos and had battles with Micro Machines.

It turned out our youngest was only afraid of one thing—dogs. So of course we started thinking about puppies. When a litter of golden retrieves was born across the road, we were hooked and had another addition to the family. My two cats tolerated it. In fact, momma cat once threw herself between "her" pup and a "wild" dog, hissing and arching her back—until it turned out that the visitor was the pup's actual mom, enthusiastic about the reunion.

The one problem in our neighborhood was an absence of other kids the right age for the boys to play with. We had to drive them everywhere. We'd decorate for Halloween with ghost lights in the bushes and carve jack-o-lanterns, but we had few trick-or-treaters. We'd have to drive the kids into town to trick-or-treat in the mall. Once when we did this, and left out candy on the doorstep with a sign saying "take one", my cat added another treat to the box—a nice juicy mouse. I have no idea if any neighbors came around and saw it before we got back—hate to think what they would have thought of us though! So what we had to do was bring Halloween to us, and we'd have dozen-kid sleep-over Halloween parties. Lynda and I would rig up a haunted house for them to run through and outdoor scavenger hunts for them in the dark. We had great fun.

We built a happy home for the boys and ourselves. Then, Hepatitis entered our lives.

5

Vanishing Wife

	Winter	Spring	Summer	Fall
1988	(2) Engagement	(3) Wedding		
89-95	(4) Raising our Children			
1996			**(5) Swelling**	(1) Christmas
1997	**(5) Diuretics**	**(5) Dehydrated**	**(5) Encephalopathy**	**(5) Encephalopathy**
1998	**(5) Encephalopathy**	**(5) Encephalopathy**	**(5) On the List**	

Hepatitis simply means "sick liver". Lynda did not have one of the hepatitis *viruses* which cause *viral* hepatitis, but her liver was indeed sick. Normally, a liver has the capability to regenerate itself—to grow as demand on it increased or to heal itself from insult. This function is what Lynda had lost. Each insult, however slight, ratcheted her down in liver function. What she had is described as cirrhosis or scarring of the liver (not to be confused with *alcoholic* cirrhosis, which specifies one particular cause out of the many possible causes), also described as "fatty infiltration" of the liver. That unfortunate description, coupled with the abdominal swelling caused Lynda to associate her condition with her life-long guilty feelings about her weight (which were at the heart of her tensions with her parents who constantly tried to make her feel awkward, fat, and inferior).

Slapped in the face by the liver disease, and having no constructive way to respond, Lynda took dieting to a new level—she basically stopped eating unless she had to. Anything she ate made her think of her liver disease and made her sick. In essence the pounds were scared off of her. While the doctors were giving her diuretics and hormone suppressants to control the fluid, Lynda dropped from pleasingly plump to skeletally thin. This is NOT a recommended diet plan! When people she knew didn't even recognize her any more and asked how she "did it", she said "You don't want to do it the way I did!"

So effective was the not-eating strategy in controlling her weight that she actually beat the doctors in the effort to dry her out. This in turn had a negative effect on her psychological problem, since the weight loss actually made the abdominal swelling more pronounced. Waitresses in restaurants would approach and ask when the baby was due. When told that Lynda was not pregnant they wouldn't believe her and would carry on about their own child-bearing experiences. Even telling them bluntly that Lynda's shape was the result of a medical problem would only slow them down a little—they would still retreat with dark looks of disbelief. Understandably, Lynda did not enjoy going out any more, and wanted to stop altogether. Swimming in public was another joy gone from her life.

But steadily, remorselessly, the diuretics and the low salt intake did their job, slowly pumping off the fluid.

What happened next should in hindsight have been predictable, but medicine is an art at best, and we had no warning. Lynda, already vanishing on a physical level, first began to vanish on another level.

Of course we all know what dieting does to the disposition. The mother of all diets caused the mother of all sour-puss attitudes. There was a lot of tension between us in those days. I was cross at her because she was cross at everybody, and given my compulsive nature, I was prone to criticize her over minor issues of planning and executing in our busy family lives. To put it more bluntly, she was distracted as Hell and seemed even more of a ding-bat than any sit-com character. That's how I felt, anyway, but knew she had good cause, and I just bit down my anger and tried to cope.

Things really got crazy one morning when she called me at work, saying that she had a flat tire; could I come fix it for her? I asked about using AAA, and she said her phone battery was dead. How was she calling me then? She had to walk into a nearby business and didn't have the AAA number with her—she was only a couple miles away—couldn't I just come rescue her?

Okay, biting the bullet I drove out to where she was. The right rear tire rim had a 2-3 inch triangular notch in it. Lynda thought maybe she hit something is all she could say, so I got out the spare tire and changed it, wondering as I worked what other damage had been done. It was a hot morning and sweat rolled off of me as Lynda just stood there and watched while I finished up. Then I looked around at the rest of the car. The front right tire was also flat with the wheel rim damaged in the same way, and Lynda hadn't realized that she had *two* flat tires on that side—just stood there in plain view of the other flat tire and watched me fix the first one of them. Amazing. Of course the car was still not drivable.

I looked back in the road to find the hubcaps and see what she had hit. The road was semi-limited-access with an off/on ramp combo separated by a cement curb. She had apparently drifted over into the turn lane and hit the protruding curb at 60 miles an hour—which explained the damage to the wheel rims. Amazing! I'm surprised that the air bag didn't blow!

So, we worked out another plan. Lynda would take my car, drop me at work, head to the University (1/2 hour away in the next town) and return to take care of the car. She would get AAA to tow it to the dealer for repairs. She seemed on top of what she needed to do, and so we parted ways.

About 4:00 I got a call from her saying she had to go to another place besides the dealer to get the rims replaced, and they were working on them now. She wasn't sure how long it would take to get it done and didn't know if she'd be able to get me before the YMCA after-school program closed, and she had to get the boys. She hadn't gotten the workers to estimate how long it would take, but we had until about 5:30 to get the boys. It seemed to me there would be a good chance of getting me first. Either way I wanted to get both cars that evening and not have to shuffle cars in the morning. I tried to propose that she pick me up first if she got done quickly enough or to get the boys first if it was that late when they got done with the wheels. This didn't make sense to her, and when I pressed her she got irritable and angry sounding—she just wanted me to be ready to go when she got there, because she'd be in a hurry to go on and get the boys. So, I thought, she wants me to sit outside my work waiting? I backed down and agreed to wait outside for her.

At 4:30 I closed up my desk and parked myself on the sidewalk outside to wait by the front door of the building, book in hand. 4:45 came—5:00 and friends and coworkers are heading home and inquire if I need a ride. I say "No thanks, I have one (I think)" and we laugh. 5:15 and a late-departing friend stops to chat, wanting to make sure I really do have a ride. 5:30 and Lynda comes down the road, pulls into the circle in front of the building, loops around the flagpole once and drives off again. She doesn't see me jumping and waving. My friend drives after her and tries to get her attention at the stop light, but she doesn't know him and gives him a dark look. Okay, fine. She realized she was late to get the boys and changed plans in mid drive. I'll wait for the round trip. I call over to the YMCA (which took a lot of calls to track down their cell phone number and get in touch with them)—and low and behold there is no Lynda there.

We wait on both ends, and we wait. All the workers at the Y have gone home except for one supervisor who has our children. Eventually, she offers to bring the boys to me and give us all a lift home. I gratefully accept, believing that Lynda has had more car trouble or an accident. It's almost 8 o'clock that night when we finally pull in to our driveway and lo and behold—there is Lynda sitting in the car in the driveway, somehow pointed back out at the road, engine off, just sitting there.

We go and see if she's okay, which she is, except for thick slurred speech, saying also that she couldn't operate the key or door or something.

We wave to the supervisor, call out our thanks to her, and she starts to back out the driveway, and Lynda panics, points at the other car, and says, "It's *moving! Stop!*"

"Yes, yes, Lynda, everything is okay," we say and wave the startled supervisor off again—and again Lynda panics as the other car begins to move, but we calm her down. We get her out of the car, and she sways as she stands. She looks and sounds like she's drunk, but she almost never drinks and didn't really have an opportunity today. Heck, she couldn't get herself out of the car and into the house!

I try to get her to go up to the bedroom and lie down, but she insists on fawning over the kids, telling them that everything is going to be all right, and of course the more she puts on a show like this for them, swaying and speaking with a slur, the more worried they get.

I know Lynda was doing all this stuff with diuretics and remembered how hot the day had been. Lynda was rushing around outside, and had probably skipped meals and maybe had had no liquids at all. Rather than being drunk, perhaps she was badly dehydrated. I finally got her to agree to drink something, but she would only touch it to her lips and then set it down. I told her if she couldn't drink I had no choice but to take her into the emergency room. She said no need; just let her rest for four hours and she would be fine. Why four hours, I asked? Where did that figure come from? That finally punched a hole in her façade, and she agreed that maybe she was a bit confused and should go see a doctor. I called a neighbor to stay with the kids (got their mother, whom I had never met, but she was willing), and off Lynda and I went to the ER together, yet again. She tried to say something to the neighbors, but the most complex sentence she could complete was "Thank you". About that time we got a call from another friend of ours, an old college chum of Lynda's and godmother of our children, informally, who we all called Auntie. I told her the problem and asked if she could hop a plane and come help, and she said "yes—be there soon".

Anyway I got Lynda to the ER and went through the check-in procedure. The routine of course even then was sit and wait, give some blood, sit and wait, and so on. I nearly lost her in the Ladies Room.

I watched as Lynda gradually lost all speech except for little sophisticated catch phrases she would use automatically, more expressions of emotion really than pieced together words. "Well, that may be…", or "Why in the world…", or "Why don't we just…", or "You really ought to…", or "Oh really. You may think that…" Almost used as a single word with full normal orchestration of voice and mannerisms. These phrases, used to influence other people and get her way, were coming out of her from a lower level than from that which it took to make a complete sentence. These were second nature to her; I never listened to her use them again without being reminded of this. There was something very disturbing about seeing one's wife dehumanized like this.

Slowly she lost even that much speech as she went into grooming behaviors, endlessly sweeping her hair back into a pony tail, over and over again, like a squirrel. This was a real problem since she would just get her hair tangled up in the IV catheter they had put in her wrist. After all the trouble they had sticking the needle in her, I didn't want to lose the IV line, so I sat there holding her hands down waiting for the doctors. By 11:00 they started giving her fluids, and by midnight she was completely comatose. Only thirteen hours earlier she had convinced me she was just being stupid over the flat tire. Eight hours earlier she had appeared to be just a bit dense on the phone. Four hours earlier she had appeared drunk, and now she was totally gone.

By morning she was established in a regular hospital room, IV's dripping, and I had had a chance to talk with the doctors. Lynda had indeed become dehydrated. The body starts burning protein. The waste products of burning the protein are generically called "ammonia" (used as an indicator for the entire class of compounds) and are the toxin that in this case impaired brain function. A normal liver converts "ammonia" into water-soluble urea, which is handled nicely by the kidneys, but Lynda's liver was not normal. Ammonia is what kills the fish in an over-crowded aquarium, smallest first. But no, this is not a permanent condition in humans—mental function is such a higher process that it is easily disrupted and is the first thing to go. The entire process could be reversed by flushing the ammonia out of her system, which would take a few days, but after which she would be herself again. There was no mortal danger except for the possibility of aspirating vomit into the lungs and getting pneumonia. Of course she had been at major risk of having an automobile accident earlier in the evening, or falling down stairs, or something of that nature. At this point, the doctors did not discuss with me the long-term implications of why this had happened, or what it foreshadowed.

Lynda was sleeping normally by morning, so I returned to the house, thanked the neighbor, got the kids off to school, and returned to the hospital to find "Auntie" there, just in from the airport—the cavalry had arrived! I went off to eat a big Chinese buffet for early lunch and shook like a leaf—then headed home for a nap, while Auntie stayed with Lynda at the hospital.

This was our first encounter with what is called "encephalopathy" which just means sick brain function. Lynda never remembered anything that happened that day. She didn't have a clue where her car was, so I had to call around a bunch of places to find it, and pay the workers involved.

Obviously we adjusted her diuretics, but still it was a balancing act from then on. Too little and she started to swell up again. Too much and she ran the risk of dehydration and encephalopathy. And of course any change in her fluid or salt intake, and any change in even the weather (and the resultant change in fluid loss to sweat etc.) would alter the balance. We learned to look for the early signs—shaking hands for instance or the inability to remember the word for something. The answer was always to push fluids.

Two medications were also prescribed. One was Lactulose, which is an indigestible sugar, basically a laxative. However, in Lynda's case she reacted strongly to it and either got nothing at low doses or immediately got runs and cramps at slightly higher doses. This level was of course counter-productive, as diarrhea contributed to the dehydration and ammonia build-up.

The other medication was Neomycin, an older antibiotic with a few side effects (nephrotoxic) that basically changed the ecology of the flora and fauna in the gut so as to shift the pH slightly more acidic. This increased the carrying power of her feces because that was the only way left to her to get rid of the ammonia—via bowel movements.

We had quite a few wobbles but no more crashes for the rest of that year. Slowly Lynda worked through all the tests that were required and eventually became officially listed as a prospective Liver Transplant Candidate in August of 98—about 2 years after the first undeniable symptoms.

Now it was time to just hunker down, hold on, and wait for that liver. Waiting list time averaged over a year and a half. How sick would she have to get before a liver came?

6

Diamonds of Despair

	Winter	Spring	Summer	Fall
1988	(2) Engagement	(3) Wedding		
89-95	(4) Raising our Children			
1996			(5) Swelling	(1) Christmas
1997	(5) Diuretics	(5) Dehydrated	(5) Encephalop-athy	(5) Encephalop-athy
1998	(5) Encephalop-athy	(5) Encephalop-athy	(5) On the List	**(6) Holding onto Family**
1999	**(6) Holding onto Family**			

Chronic pain is the worst kind, because it wears away at your soul and makes you a person you are not proud to be.

My personal acquaintance with chronic pain came from knee problems. I was not light weight, and the building in which I worked had several stories connected by stairwells with half-flight runs of concrete steps. Always in a hurry, I would rush up or down these steps.

Imagine the stresses involved when a 250 plus pound man runs down a half-flight of steps, lands on one leg for a twisting turn into the next run of steps. My knee couldn't take the pressure. The initial pain was short and sharp. The aftermath took three years to work through. I would shift the way I walked to favor the injured side of the knee to avoid twisting it the wrong way. The knee would get better, but I was using unfamiliar muscles, so I'd get cramps. That in turn changed the way I walked, so I'd put into play a different set of muscles and end up with back pain. And so on. Eventually, everything would stop hurting (I developed a limp), and I'd get going too fast again and re-injure the knee.

On and on this went for three years, and I know now how cross I can get with friends and family when I'm in chronic pain.

The only doctor I visited wanted to leap right in to arthroscopic surgery before really trying anything else, and I never went back to him. Instead, my folkdance leader suggested leg lifts to strengthen the muscle that runs down the front of the leg, and prevents the buckling of the knee. This is in fact what did the trick for me.

I've also had lower back trouble as a young adult—probably didn't get enough exercise. That was bad, but at worst a pinched nerve only ran to a couple days on my back. The knee was worse because of the cascade of muscular-skeletal adjustments that just transferred the pain from place to place.

Later, when I had to cope on separate occasions with heel-spurs (really too much weight on poorly made shoes) and with a damaged joint in my foot from a soccer injury, I was less prone to despair and cussedness, because I had some perspective on what it would take to deal with this sort of injury. It took a whole year for my foot joint to heal, and the pain finally to depart.

All this gave me perspective for understanding Lynda's turn with chronic pain.

Over the course of six to twelve months, Lynda's body fat dropped more than forty pounds, and her abdominal fluid rose sharply, and then fell slowly. This continuously adjusted her balance and posture, and soon every muscle in her back was screaming full time. At the worst point, her abdomen was so swollen that the actual wall muscles hurt from being so stretched.

So it was no surprise that Lynda became progressively more cranky and cross and finally could only think of her back most of the time.

The back rubs that used to be a shared joy became a necessity for her and a chore for me. It was not easy or reasonable for me to expect reciprocation. For me to simply say I was tired would turn into a pissing match over who was *more* tired—not exactly a productive activity. Suffice it to say that I got very little sympathy for my problems as long as hers were bigger.

This was a rough time for our relationship—not just because of the pain-drain. After the first big episode of encephalopathy, the functioning of the family was threatened by the possibility of a recurrence. I was often put in the position of noticing symptoms before Lynda either noticed or admitted them, and was having to push her into taking the proper steps: drink, drink, drink! As much as the whole thing was tied up with dehydration and bowel movements, we managed to get by without digging to that level of humiliation for her, and kept the encephalopathy at bay.

And yet, this period certainly shook Lynda up a lot. The most obvious manifestation was her dreams. Lynda would wake me up at night by screaming in her dreams because people were chasing her with knives. I took it to be an obvious manifestation of her fear of surgery, which she spoke about as if someone was going to "make" her go through it.

I couldn't convince her that the surgeons were trying to help her—she didn't want to have to have surgery and still didn't believe, bottom line, that it was necessary. When you realize that delays at this stage, for instance avoiding scheduling tests, cause delays in getting officially on the transplant list, you realize that this fear was indirectly hurting her chances of a successful outcome in the liver surgery. That didn't matter though. Lynda had to deal with her self-image and had to *want* the surgery before it could happen.

One doctor put it well in saying that a transplant is major surgery with serious risks and serious quality of life impact post surgery. They would not perform a transplant unless this was the best choice available. This leads to the unhappy but realistic conclusion that Lynda would have to get pretty sick before she would be wanting the surgery to come. Later, she would ask, just how sick would she have to get before a liver was made available for her? Her perspective slowly shifted from "What if they do?" to "What if they don't?" Lynda knew that the only way to get to the other side was through a very dark period in the middle, where she was sick enough to be ready for a liver, but on tenterhooks waiting for it to come. That time may or may not be spent laid up in the hospital.

With that kind of cloud hanging over one's head, life takes on a new urgency and a new focus. Staying focused on things that really matter became an imperative, and Lynda threw herself into her work with a sort of desperation. Although it gave her an outlet, something constructive to do with all that negative energy, it also exhausted her.

Our tenth anniversary came and highlighted the dependence Lynda felt on my help. For the first time she became clinging and insecure and little touches of romance took on a far deeper level of significance. I made sure that flowers often appeared in our house in those days (usually in the hands of little boys). Eventually Lynda fixated on the issue of the diamond ring she hadn't wanted on our engagement. What was then disdained in an arrangement between partners became a symbol of security for her.

She joined me at a technical conference in California, and we stopped in the San Francisco bay area to select a fancy diamond ring that few newlyweds could afford. We agreed that some day we'd spend a similar amount on my fantasy—a home computer system to top them all. The trip was marred only by her attempt to go on a sight-seeing drive that left her hot and panicky after being lost without a map for most of a day. She refused to recognize any limits her condition placed on her activities! We took custody of the ring on the way back to the airport, and returned to Appalachia.

It was a time of loneliness and adjustment for me. Although neither of us was willing to admit it, I lost a partner during this period, and gained a dependant. Our good years were gone, and not only did I feel more alone than I had ever been since leaving home for college as a single young man, I now had serious responsibilities of family to carry.

It was during this period that I flopped between my various hobbies, trying to recall joys gone by, and eventually began a journal which would serve me well in the years ahead.

Journal Entry, April 23, 1999.

As my life goes by, I have often thought about capturing the high points, or keeping a log. We'll see if this effort is more successful than in the past. "Why?" we will explore on these pages, but it feels different this time.

Today I was reading a Dilbert book at lunch. Chinese being bad for my weight at 260 pounds and fighting off a new round of undercarriage problems, I opted to settle for the fortune cookie as dessert. For perhaps the first time in my life, I was so wrapped up in the book and worried about time to head back to work, that I completely ignored the fortune. Minutes later, I realized this and picked it out of the sauce on my plate. It read "You will not be distracted from your goals." A self-referential fortune cookie?

Yesterday, ants joined an organizational meeting I was running, and began exploring the overhead projector. The humans in the room were grossly (pun) outnumbered. I've been reading a lot about ants and their diversity and was greatly amused. Ants have dominated our ecosystem virtually unchanged since before Dinosaurs. A typical colony has thirty times the number of neurons as in the human brain.

I'm concerned about my younger son. I had put a lot of faith into Scouts as an institution for developing boys, but it's not turning out to be his "thing". Instead, soccer seems to be his love. If I can do anything for him, it will include supporting that, so now I'm being drawn into organized sports—I who have always disdained such. I may even get a professional "E" license to coach!

My older son is on a competitive soccer team but seems less in love with it—though he does like Scouts. Part of it was the job I've done as his cub scout Den Leader, but I was not able to do that for the younger one (and what a disaster his den turned out to be!) But my eldest will be "moving up" to Boy Scouts middle of next year—it's a race to see which boy is "out" of cubs first.

My eldest is missing tomorrow's pack meeting because of soccer, so never made a Rain gutter Regatta boat. My younger son never wanted to make one—and is ending up at a friend's house tonight for birthday party and thus not going to pack meeting tomorrow morning either. I find myself, as assistant cub master and den leader, committed to going without either!

I agreed to pay $70 for a set of yellow practice jerseys today.

I spent an hour today with our new accountant—this makes two motorcycle-riding accountants I've known at work now. Must be a reaction to the work they do or something.

◆   ◆   ◆

Journal Entry, April 29, 1999.

Today's fortune cookie (can't keep away from the Chinese food) was opened one-handed in the car while rushing to an outlying building for a Business Unit team meeting. The fortune: "You are traveling in the right direction." How reassuring! It actually turned out to be a pretty upbeat meeting for a change.

◆   ◆   ◆

Journal Entry, April 30, 1999.

Stood up for the cause of Enlightenment today in a Sales meeting—they showed us prototype rating system for the field guys—ranking categories is fine for identifying development opportunities, but this thing weighted the categories and gave a final total score. Result of that would be infighting, paranoia, and demoralization. The Employee Development System and Company Way is to take the people we have and develop them into the best performers and the best team players that we can. This new system flies in the face of that enlightened corporate policy, and I made no bones about pointing it out.

◆   ◆   ◆

Journal Entry, May 6, 1999.

Yesterday I ate Chinese again—can't keep away. The salt gives me an immediate two pound boost in weight, but given the veggie content I'm not sure how it comes out after the salt peak dies off.

Anyway, there I am thinking about the fact that I'm recording my fortune cookies in this journal and the increased importance they are given thereby. This one read "You like sports, horses, and gambling, but not in excess." Boy did this one miss the target—I still recall the horse ride which ended up with me kissing the dirt at age seven, and I hadn't ridden again for at least twenty years. I hadn't gambled for money since my father and grandfather tried to teach me about poker (I won but saw from their horror-stricken faces how important they thought the lesson). I don't consider the $20 I sacrificed to blackjack on our honeymoon cruise to be gambling either—just expensive entertainment to say I'd done it. The only saving grace for this Chinese fortune cookie was the ambiguous interpretation allowed by the word "excess", which is of course the Rorschach ink-blot basis for much of fortune telling. It recalls to me the "perverse spirit" idea from my youth—the idea that the instant you try to harness or rely on a psychic power or fortune telling device, it turns against you out of spiteful perversion (to maintain the mystery of its existence, of course!) Being the "victim" of such ironic perversion always brought a smile to my face then, as this fortune cookie did now. Magic only works if it can avoid the lime-light of cold rational measurements—but there is *always* room for the snake-oil charlatan, the dishonest artist or scientist angling for a grant, or the wishful thinkers of the world to wiggle out of anything. These things work, or not, depending on your *belief*. Strength of "faith" and religion can of course work the same way—great as long as you don't analyze them too closely.

I'm listening to the sad/triumphant/human/ephemeral music from Titanic. The mood of it really resonates with me these days—what with Lynda's medical condition capping everything off.

She came back from the transplant center telling me that her kidneys were losing the battle to handle enough medication to keep the fluid at bay. She must choose between carrying more fluid and being periodically (more and more frequently) incapacitated by her back problems *or* getting a shunt put in place to remove it and taking a 25% chance that she'll experience some amount of encephalopathy. Thus she would basically lose her self in a mental fog of encephalopathy until the liver transplant comes. She's done so well in avoiding that soul-rending problem since the neomycin shifted the pH of her gut. Now enters the risk that she could have *permanent* damage to her kidneys after transplant if they keep the medicine too high for too long. What a choice—between torture and loss of self/dignity—what a classic dilemma!

All these factors are reasons for writing this journal. I've taken some tentative moves towards learning more about counseling options for myself—same deal.

I was amused to find a book, physically just like this one, in which I had planned to record monographs on subjects technical, philosophical, and sociological. I've started lots of writing projects over the years, but always lost a sense of purpose. I have to laugh at myself for the cockiness of some of the projects.

This time though, sense of purpose turned out to be the least of my worries.

◆   ◆   ◆

7

The Big Crash

	Winter	Spring	Summer	Fall
1988	(2) Engagement	(3) Wedding		
89-95	(4) Raising our Children			
1996			(5) Swelling	(1) Christmas
1997	(5) Diuretics	(5) Dehydrated	(5) Encephalop-athy	(5) Encephalop-athy
1998	(5) Encephalopa-thy	(5) Encephalopa-thy	(5) On the List	(6) Holding to Family
1999	(6) Holding to Family	**(7) Big Crash, Shunt**		

Journal Entry, May 19, 1999.

What a weekend! Lynda is in the hospital with complications from liver disease.

Thursday the 13th of May, Lynda was on a business trip to Red Boiling Springs, population about six thousand. The pressure on her portal vein that feeds the liver had built up enough that blood had engorged the veins that line the esophagus. These started bleeding in a number of places called "varicosities"—varicose veins that then bled into her esophagus. This drained into her stomach with the result that she vomited blood.

She called me at the house and had me get in touch with her doctor's answering service, it being evening. They said go immediately to the nearest emergency room, which was an hour and a half away in the big city. They said don't drive, get an ambulance! They stabilized her in the hospital there, and I spent Friday morning trying to figure whether to go 4-5 hours one direction to where she was or 4-5 hours in the other direction to her transplant center. Eventually, Friday pm. I headed to the transplant center—Lynda beat me by half an hour, since she took an air ambulance.

One small episode of bloody vomitius occurred Thursday night at the first big city hospital, another just before I got to the transplant center, and a fourth *major* one just after I got there (I held the bucket for her—she lost about a pint on that one).

So, Friday night the transplant center got to do another endoscopy and put rubber bands on the weak spots and added clotting factors to stop the bleeding.

Saturday she was pretty lucid—but liquid diet only plus IV's. She beat me at cards.

Sunday she entered the zone—combination of benedryl, morphine, other pain killer, and beginning to digest the blood she swallowed—she went encephalopathic. Pretty much missed Monday morning too. But, she had picked up thirty pounds of fluid since Thursday, and she started having pain. Monday night was a night from Hell—she was miserable and fought everybody; neither of us got any sleep.

Tuesday they drew nine pounds of fluid off her abdomen with a needle and discovered that she had serious infections—it had even spread to her bloodstream. They got her antibiotics, but the pain was pretty severe. They eventually got her a body-length water-circulating hot pad and enough pain killer to make an elephant fly. Wednesday afternoon (now as I write this) she's high as a kite.

This weekend perhaps the infection will be clear, and they can proceed with placing a *shunt*—which will help with the problems with back pain, fluid, cramped digestive tract, and most of all—the possibility of another potentially fatal bleed!

◆   ◆   ◆

I finished reading a story (was it Saturday?) in which the color blue figured prominently in saving a space colony. On the back of today's fortune (yep, Chinese food again—this time with pot stickers and plum wine) it said "Learn Chinese—Blue = Lan-Se". Hmmm. The actual fortune was "you will inherit some money or a small piece of land". At the time I thought of my recently deceased Grandmother, not Lynda, but later in the day I made the connection and was glad to discover that I wasn't on a morbid track with Lynda. This afternoon my Dad called with offers of assistance, including paying back some old loans as soon as my Grandmother's will goes through probate. Connections abound...Then today's fortune cookie—"Reach out and give someone a supportive hand". This should be called an imperative cookie.

Played "Fish" and "Old Maid" with the eleven year old daughter of some of Lynda's colleagues in the area, while they visited in the hospital. There's a girl full of energy! She had a lot of spirit, and despite being a bit of a Tomboy, and pitching for her softball team, she insisted that Star Wars Episode I was a boy's movie, and she wasn't interested.

◆   ◆   ◆

Journal Entry, Sunday, May 23, 1999—

The Day it All Cut Loose—recorded after the fact of course.

They'd been fighting the infection pretty hard, but this was at the expense of the kidneys. Saturday they put her on dopamine drip to open up the veins to her kidneys. She went through the night fine, but acidosis set in Sunday about 9-10 am. She developed heart arrhythmia and very labored breathing. Things got very busy for awhile. They got permission to intubate her if necessary. They got permission to do electro shock jumpstart on her heart if needed—this made her eyes go very wide. Her pulse was skipping beats and wandered from 30 to 50 per minute. Her blood pressure was good though, unlike the low of 58/33 we saw during the infection. I found out later that dopamine actually raises blood pressure, while risking making it erratic.

She ended up in the respiratory ICU with an ECG down into her heart chamber and a major tap into femoral vein for dialysis. Sunday was very touchy and I "sent up the balloon" asking grandparents to come be with the kids back home and suggesting that Auntie and Lynda's relatives from out west come now...

Monday the dialysis did a great job stabilizing her.

Auntie and I went to the local Chinese restaurant with the tremendous buffet while Lynda's folks visited. My fortune read "All the news you receive will be positive and uplifting."

Upon our return we learned that the infection was clear, and that her priority was being bumped up to a 2A, which means the next type O (Rh irrelevant) liver is *hers*! Sixty-five type O's were transplanted by this facility last year. The wait ought to be less than a week—especially with Memorial Day and expected traffic fatalities coming up.

◆   ◆   ◆

I should take a little time to describe the facility Lynda had chosen. In looking over the different places across the country that did transplants, Lynda wanted one that was big enough to be well experienced with the procedures, but small enough to still pay special attention to the needs of the individual. This may have been most important to her—choosing a place where she would be treated like an individual. She chose a program at a university medical school and I could never fault them for the care and attention they gave to either of us—patient or spouse. The university town provided some interesting things to see and places to eat when we were not in the hospital. But it was still a big place, with all the friendly people trying their best to compensate for the impersonality and inefficiency of the institution. For the most part they stayed ahead of it, and we greatly appreciated their efforts. Each patient's circumstances are unique and I never blamed our outcomes on anyone who cared for Lynda. Everyone was so clearly doing their best.

◆   ◆   ◆

Journal Entry, June 5, 1999.

It had been a long nine days waiting. Sometime during that time I got a Chinese fortune saying, "The small steps you take will ultimately bring you great fortune". I saved it but don't think I was greatly inspired. I was pretty tired. Lynda was fighting with muscular discomfort from the prolonged bed rest—back, hip, and legs. I did a lot of rubbing. Since all the pain killers and muscle relaxants clear through the Liver, they had to play a balancing act and were constantly adjusting dosage and trying one-time things they couldn't repeat. Lynda said they were torturing her, and she was reduced to begging in tears for relief. Other days they would just give her morphine.

Thursday, a liver came available. We were all very excited and on a high—Lynda somewhat anxious of course. The surgeons headed off to "harvest" the liver. To relieve the tension, we tried to remember the words to "Amazing Grace", sang, and fidgeted.

They got her asleep and into the Operating Room before they decided the liver was bad and aborted the surgery.

So, they wheeled her off to the recovery room where the horror began.

They give a patient sedatives and anesthesia to put her asleep, plus a paralytic agent to stop her muscles from moving (and put a tube down her throat to control breathing mechanically).

Well, the sedative wore off before the paralysis drug. This was due to a combination of factors—the normal 15-20 minutes for the paralytic was greatly extended, because it clears through the liver (Duh!) plus they have no EEG in the recovery room to monitor brain function, as they do in the operating room.

Lynda was conscious but had eyes taped shut and was unable to move or signal in any way. The people around her did not know she was aware and spoke very loosely, one nursing student calling her "the liver" and talked about going home. Lynda had no idea what was going on and whether something had gone wrong with the sedative—she thought they might be about to cut into her and she had no way to tell them she was aware of everything. Also they kept administering electric shocks—torture as far as she could tell, though really designed to test for motor function which they must have before they can take her off the mechanical breathing. When she did regain motor function, a male nurse was a big comfort (I was not allowed in yet), but she didn't know anyone. None of the liver team that had made all the promises was there.

In short, Lynda was traumatized, was shaking like a leaf and vowed she'd kill herself before she'd let them take her back to the OR. Obviously we've got *lots* to work on now. I understand this experience was actually a punishment used by voodoo priests in the Caribbean, drugging the culprit into paralysis while he could hear the villagers all around him—the origin of the zombie mythos.

I was angry of course, and knew that this sort of thing formed a very firm basis for a lawsuit—or threat of one at least. This experience coupled with the poor and erratic pain management plus you could argue she came in defended by antibiotics as a customary response to the threat of infection—a *known* risk. The antibiotics were terminated for her first 4-5 days opening the door for the infection which she developed—which was life threatening and led to the sequence bed-rest/immobile/muscular pains/torture of inadequate pain killer.

I spent the morning (early through lunch) planning how to apply leverage. I wanted it to be constructive so needed to know where to push and what to ask for. I waited, trying to make contact with some of Lynda's local colleagues with connections to the hospital system to consult before doing something dumb.

After lunch, a chaplain finally spread the word about our situation, and people began to show up in droves—many sympathetic but some to cover ass. (Lynda and the anesthesiologist had very different priorities for the recovery room—he was rather self-righteous about the job he had done and his responsibility to keep her alive regardless of comfort). We were visited by Patient Relations, Risk Management (Legal), the Chaplain, a Rabbi, 1-2 psychologists, the transplant coordinator, the surgeon, another doctor from the liver team, the attending physicians, the head nurse...I think we'll get what we need, if we can just figure out what that is. An EEG in the recovery room next time for sure.

Lynda has a rough road ahead, and a very big challenge to rise to, in facing the OR again.

◆   ◆   ◆

Journal Entry, June 11, 1999.

I'm having a hard time reconstructing the time sequences here, but the next fortune cookie was a duplicate of the previous—about small steps ultimately leading to great things.

At the time I was a bit amused because I had just written about not "getting it" the first time around. I went days wanting to write about the duplicate—now that I read my previous entry I'm even more confused about timing and have to smile at my mental state.

Lynda has been coping with the extreme trauma of her paralytic experience. To add to that, a twisted ankle inflamed old injuries (bone break and an arthritic spot) thus making her immobile in bed again—at risk of another fall. She kept saying, "What next?"

The "next" made me feel like she'd run out of new things—Thursday June 10, at 5:00 am., I got called to say she was bleeding again, from both ends.

So endoscopy #3 at this hospital was indicated. However, this time it was worse. Her blood pressure fell to 57/16—I didn't think it could go so low. This was obviously a very serious bleed. They couldn't *both* give her meds to raise her blood pressure (dopamine) *and* sedate her for the endoscopy to band off the bleeds. So they decided we needed an emergency "TIPS shunt" to partially bypass the liver and take the pressure off. They called me in to help two psychologists with the very difficult task of getting her consent, as she had indicated that she would not go through with the TIPS. She was very clear that she did *not* want to die but apparently wanted to argue about the options available (none). Ultimately she relented and agreed to the procedure. For the record, the following day she was sure that she did *not* have a shunt in place, so must have been under the influence of *something* during that conversation.

Anyway the procedure (an "intrusive radiology" in that they enter through the jugular and pulmonary artery) was Thursday from 2:30—6:30. She came out with a breathing tube.

No MD anesthesiologist was on hand during the "procedure"—two nurses only—and the result was they had set her up for a repeat of paralysis without sedative—this time for an hour and a half! I asked questions, discovered the situation, and insisted they sedate her or send in the doctor to talk with me—and got the amnesia drug. All our preparation of the liver team and the anesthesia crew and the administration was almost for nothing—this procedure was done by the *vascular* people, who were not in the loop. Aaargh!

Anyway, I spent 13 hours Thursday night with Lynda as she gradually woke up and eventually came off the breathing tube—with her frustrated and fighting all the way.

At about 8:30 she was talking and wanted to be left alone, so I cut out for breakfast and a 4-hour nap.

On my return I found out that she had half-pulled out the catheter in her jugular vein and lost a lot of blood—still fighting the docs and having to be restrained. Really gave the nurses a scare.

She was already encephalopathic from digesting all the blood she had swallowed—it took me five minutes to convince her of the plumbing arrangements (two catheters so she didn't need to go to the bathroom).

Eventually, "atovan" took the edge off so she could sleep, so now I'm coming in to sleep too.

On the way down to the "motel" room (some cots they rent out in the basement) I caught a view I had never seen before until this our four-week anniversary at the hospital. Visible only through a diagonal glass pane at the curve of the passage is a long view of a fairy-tower rising above the misty landscape (possibly water vapor rising from the cooling units of the hospital after a rainy day?). The tower is the campus clock tower, I guess, but it was quite incongruous to see in the midst of the old-paint utilitarian hospital setting.

Reminded me of the bizarre precipitate I got in a test tube back in graduate school that I thought was the spitting image of a gnome sitting in "thinker" position on a mushroom—my previous incongruous fantasy vision after a long, fatiguing ordeal in the lab. Sort of like Indians that starved themselves as part of a rite of passage and had visions…

Reminder—to write about the two extremes of "equipment guy" I saw recently. One was one of the construction workers who depend on metal snaphooks for safety lines, who walk around dragging these life-saving devices behind them on the concrete, bouncing at the end of the tethers, with no concern for the damage they're doing to them, and the consequent risk to their lives. The other was the guy bringing in a gas fitting for a breathing treatment to Lynda's room. I asked what it was for and he said he was "just an equipment guy", obviously taking psychological refuge in this identity to avoid getting sucked into the pain and human misery he saw around him on a routine basis. Such an interesting identification with pride in what he did, while avowing total ignorance of what the equipment was used for!

Well, I guess I just did write about them. Real juxtaposition of attitudes—insight into characters for writing some day.

I've started reading Carl Sagan's "the Daemon Haunted World", about people turning from science to superstition in the modern world.

◆   ◆   ◆

Journal Entry, June 18, 1999.

Despite the Doctors saying that she'd be encephalopathic for days, until midweek probably, she popped right out of it Sunday morning in good spirits, strong and stable.

The docs are amazed at the recuperative powers she's displaying. She doesn't remember any of it—the time between the 3rd endoscopy and the shunt (our trying to get agreement to do the TIPS shunt) <u>or</u> the 13 hours after with the breathing tube—a definite mercy.

Today is the five-week anniversary of being admitted here. Twenty four days without a good liver would be four standard deviations out on the Poisson distribution—a pretty improbable event. Lynda's getting well enough for the Doctors to discuss moving her out of the ICU/Critical Care system—which might then drop her priority on the transplant waiting list. Not a good thing to contemplate.

I'm of course starting to get antsy about work what with a boss change and bits and pieces from the field about my new materials and how they did or did not perform. I really don't think I'll have the patience to go back to the same job situation again. I think I'll go to the VP and lay it on the line—if you've got no use for somebody who can "make things happen", then I need to be applying for more traditional leadership roles. Specifically ask him to approve my application for a Supervisor slot.

I look at myself these days—getting my eight hours of sleep but still very tired. I think this is characteristic of my way of dealing with stress and crisis—rock steady in the crunch, but then it catches up with me later. I think it's catching up with me now. I feel like I have a lot to write about—garnered some more perspective about what is worth telling.

I also saw "The Phantom Menace" yesterday. What a thrill to be back in my teen years again, seeing a brand-new Star Wars come onto the big screen for the first time. I was grinning from ear to ear after that.

◆   ◆   ◆

Journal Entry, June 21, 1999.

What an ironic twist. Lynda is doing *so* well they've moved her to a regular room and dropped her to a 2B priority—drastically postponing the transplant. She had invested *so* much in preparing mentally for this, convincing herself her life depended on a new liver, and that she *had* to go into the O.R. again, that the news came as a slap in the face. She wasn't going to get "her" liver, and she'll have to go through it all again.

Actually she's in better shape than in a long time. The transplant will occur in *weeks* rather than months or a year (or so it sounds like), so we can't do anything too radical with travel this summer/fall.

Looks likely we'll be going home Wednesday PM!

8

Playing Dominos

	Winter	Spring	Summer	Fall
1988	(2) Engagement	(3) Wedding		
89-95	(4) Raising our Children			
1996			(5) Swelling	(1) Christmas
1997	(5) Diuretics	(5) Dehydrated	(5) Encephalopathy	(5) Encephalopathy
1998	(5) Encephalopathy	(5) Encephalopathy	(5) On the List	(6) Holding to Family
1999	(6) Holding to Family	(7) Big Crash, Shunt	**(8) Dominos Fall**	

Journal Entry—July 6, 1999.

We've been home a couple weeks now. Coping with Lynda's Lactulose/Encephalopathy balance has been touchy. We had a wake-up call at a 4th of July picnic, when she overdid it, got dehydrated, and a touch loopy. Her attempt at steady progress in walking and climbing stairs has been interrupted by a fall and bruised tail bone. She's not supposed to drive for another week. We're going to have a housekeeper come in for four hours three times a week.

At work, I've started the Supervisor Selection etc. process application with a cover letter to my boss and the VP about my career interests. I need to revise that cover letter to emphasize teaching and vision vs. being a crutch for the Business Organization now. With that emphasis in mind, group leader isn't such an "also ran" as compared to leading a technical effort.

I really have a lot of work to do setting up patents and working up the next batch of samples for regulatory submission, not to mention technical reports to be written.

Did I mention my new boss? His appointment was announced while I was gone, and he will be taking over August first. Shook his hand once now.

◆   ◆   ◆

Journal Entry—July 14, 1999.

Yesterday ate Chinese again—hit my all time high of 270 and 1/2 pounds. My feet are killing me—I've got to go on a bread/fruit/veggie diet to get below 250 again for my feet—220 would be a major landmark, but that's longer term. Below 200 is recommended—maybe even 160 according to the actuarial tables, which I have a hard time visualizing.

Why the problem? Stress leads to eating. Direct connection. More below.

But I got an interesting fortune. "Soon you will be sitting on top of the world." My first reaction was a sarcastic "Yeah, right!"—more below. Disbelief in the fortune cookie process. There was a brief flash about new job prospects of going back to Research (Ivory Tower-> sitting on top—get it?), but then my BS detector kicked in, and I realized that all points are "top" of a gravity producing sphere, so in a sense I'm already sitting on top of the world. Cute. Makes for an interesting alien perspective snippet for a SF story some day.

Why the stress? Monday's icing on the cake was rain on top of soccer camp and messed up childcare (which pulled me out of work) but the "cake" itself was Lynda's situation.

Friday, July 9th she was unreasonably irritated with me, signaling possible encephalopathy, but I figured she was on lactulose and fixed her a 15cc dose for the morning. She was calling off her business meeting after a long hard day Thursday.

On the way home from work, I called to hear only the phone being picked up and dropped. I got the boys from a friend's house and tried to hurry home, but the main road was under construction, and we were routed the long way around. The phone was on the floor, and the controller for the hot pad was hung up in the phone cradle. Lynda swore the housekeeper never came, even though the two of them went out in the car to run errands, and she had eaten a hamburger. The GI doctor on call said if I was comfortable doing it, to ply her with lactulose and get her in to her main GI doctor on Monday.

I felt we had pretty well got things under control by Monday (hard weekend) when soccer camp was rained out. I had to return boys home after searching for the field in the rain, then attend a 10-12 business team meeting. Gave the boys to a friend and headed to Lynda's doctor. The doctor wanted to run a bunch of tests, so Lynda was admitted to the hospital for the night. Didn't know whether she would be released Tuesday—so there I was eating Chinese again between phone calls—still trying to bail out from my six-week "vacation" and get back in the groove. We did get to bring her home after (our) dinner. Thence ensued a scene involving last-minute urine catches, two runs on useless pharmacies, apple juice, fig newton's, raw hamburger left on the counter top for dinner, having the boys (both with Pink Eye) tuck themselves in, followed by me dashing to the only late-night grocery/pharmacy for a 9:35-10:05 argument with their new computer system over Blue Cross cards and the fact that there were two doctors in the book with the same last name. Ultimately the run was worth it since Lynda's foot felt so much better in the morning (we were fighting gout now too) that she walked on it without thinking! She gets to take care of the housekeeper and her medicine while I get the boys off to soccer, with sprinkles of rain in the air.

The car needs new tires and an oil change. My feet *really* hurt. I've probably got Pink Eye too. I've got a lot of work to do and not sure where to start, plus soccer and cub scout obligations. House air filter screens need washed. Thank goodness the heat pump problem turned out to be just a hose sticking up into the fan!

◆   ◆   ◆

Journal Entry—July 30th.

Well, we're back in the hospital again with serious encephalopathy. She's been fighting against taking the medications since we came back. I think I need to tabulate the low points. Auntie is coming tomorrow, probably will take care of my youngest son while I'm off to scout camp with the oldest for the weekend.

Date:	Item:
7/4	First physiological shakes etc.
7/9 Friday	Crash at end of day, to hospital
7/10-11	Home for the weekend
7/12	Day trip to the hospital, home that night
7/22 Thurs	One of Lynda's colleagues left in driveway with cell phone, unable to get Lynda to answer the door, Lynda brought to hospital, kept overnight for testing.

7/23	Brought home for weekend.
7/26 Mon	Appointment at the transplant center, she was confused in the morning, incredibly bad trip there, checked in to the ER instead of going to the appointment
7/27	Testing, getting better, discuss a plan
7/28 Wed	Heading home, Lynda convinced them that the morning's grogginess was just fatigue.
7/29	Launched into "the Plan" to care for Lynda at home, fully committed, with the tools we thought we needed to control the encephalopathy, took six times 30cc lactulose and had maybe six bowel movements but still crashed between supper and 10 pm. I stayed up with her until about 1 am, then got some sleep. She was not getting any better, so time to give up.
7/30 Fri	Here I am at the hospital E.R. again, waiting for a doctor to decide what to do.

◆   ◆   ◆

I was really at the end of my rope. I felt that the encephalopathy thing had beaten us. Out of that, though, came a glimmer of psychological relief—I was incapable of caring for Lynda by myself, so therefore I didn't have to try to shoulder the burden alone. If it came to that, Lynda could just check in to the hospital and wait there—let the professionals take care of her now.

Somehow though, I was convinced to take her home and try again, but this time, I called for help. Auntie was the first to come down, but it was Lynda's surrogate sister that did us the best turn, with her background in therapy. I gave her a list of all the friends and relatives who had offered help and asked her to figure out a plan for us. I needed to get back to work, both for my career's sake and my own sanity; I was not cut out to be a nursemaid.

Lynda's sister instead explained what a Certified Nursing Assistant or CNA was, and called around for us to see what was available in the area. A CNA has very basic training in caring for indigent people; monitoring vital signs, helping people take medicines if you meter it out for them, and so forth. She found an agency that could provide CNA's that not only could deal with the medical and nursing issues, but could also drive Lynda and the boys, and do light housekeeping in the down-time. We had been paying the YMCA to care for our children a few hours after school, so those funds could be diverted to the CNA, who could keep an eye on the kids until I got home. The best part about the agency was that if the regular CNA was ill, finding a replacement was the responsibility of the agency, so we could depend on someone always being there for Lynda.

All this came for a fraction of the cost per hour that I was having to sacrifice by missing work. The CNA's were a godsend, and life again became somewhat stable. I started out trying to hold their hours to 40 per week, with me working home some and using the CNA's to let me take the boys to soccer and scouts in the evenings. We went through a few CNA's before we found a regular that not only could handle the diverse challenges our family faced, but wanted all the work hours we could give her. She worked out so well, that I quickly resumed a full work schedule and gladly paid for the extra hours to cover special events. I got tremendous relief from having help, and no longer having to shoulder alone the hour-to-hour burden of worrying about Lynda. When Lynda started trying to flush magazines down the toilet, I simply warned the CNA that she was having a bad day and headed to work with a smile.

We thought Lynda's condition was predictable for a few hours ahead, and she still tried to drive occasionally on an errand. One day I got a call from the police who had pulled her over for driving in the turn lane and bouncing off the curbs, and that was the end of her driving. Step by step she surrendered her liberties and accepted the care of the CNA's.

Life got better for me, but for Lynda, it just drew out, longer and longer, spiraling down, as she waited for that liver to come.

◆   ◆   ◆

Journal Entry—August 18, 1999.

We took her into the hospital that last Friday in July. She came back Sunday with Auntie while my oldest boy and I went to scout camp. Lynda's surrogate sister then took the duty end of that week, for most of the next week.

This week we are starting to work with Certified Nursing Assistants (CNA's) for coverage of days, soccer practice, and scouts for our older boy.

Lynda is taking the protein restriction more seriously, and we're being more aggressive with the lactulose and the fiber, so we've kept her out of the hospital. We have had at least one episode per week of clear encephalopathy with about a six-hour or less duration. Keep those bowels moving!

I have an appointment for a physical exam on August 30th to check on weight, cholesterol, PSA baseline, heart, whatever—stress, feet…Also with a psychologist September 9th for counseling on how to deal with stress.

◆   ◆   ◆

Lynda's increased encephalopathy was only the first domino to fall after the events of that summer.

The increased encephalopathy was a very straight-forward effect. They had reduced the pressure build up on the portal vein by shunting a portion of her blood around (actually tunneling through) the liver. This did the trick of keeping her from bleeding to death, but of course her blood was no longer being 100% processed by the liver. There is a reason why the liver is there to do a job. With the shunt, all the toxins that affected the brain built up even quicker, and so we had to keep an even tighter control on fluids, protein, and medications to control the bowel movements.

I struggled to understand what was going on, and tried to "connect the dots" in the sequence of events that was being revealed to us. I saw Lynda's problems as a series of dominos falling one by one down a path. The cirrhosis increased the pressure in the portal vein, which caused the veins to leak, which caused the fluid build-up and eventual bleeding, which caused both the fluid and blood stream to become infected, which caused the encephalopathy and further lost mental function, which dictated use of strong antibiotics, which shut down her kidneys (and almost her heart)—requiring dialysis to recover. While her kidneys were shut down, uric acid built up in her blood stream to the saturation point and beyond, and began precipitating out as little crystals in her joints, particularly her big toes. This is the mechanism by which diet or kidney disease causes what is commonly called gout (or more technically gouty arthritis).

Of course this was just me trying to find explanations in order to regain some feeling of control. The opposite view is just as valid, that when one's energy reserves are overwhelmed, one loses the ability to react and everything shuts down all at once. In truth the myriad systems in the human body are inter-related in complicated ways and we will never have enough information about everything all at once, let alone how such conditions then change with time, to be able to program it all into a computer and solve the equation. Even if the day comes when we could in theory, resources will limit what we can do in real time as a matter of practice. Medicine will always remain an art.

The first soreness from the gout came right after her aborted surgery, and she assumed someone had banged her around while unconscious—one more insult to add to the pile. Her twisted ankle and other pains covered the effects of the gout such that it went unnoticed for weeks, but the seed crystals had been planted. Not until we got home and ramped up her medication to the max in an effort to deal with the encephalopathy, did her uric acid levels climb and the crystals start to grow.

The pain of gout can be awful. Some say it is the very most intense pain we can experience, and it does not desensitize you over time. She couldn't concentrate on anything due to the pain, and, as it got worse, she eventually couldn't even walk. She would have to crawl on her hands and knees to get to the bathroom. So even when she was fully possessed of her mental facilities, she was humiliated in a whole new fashion.

Of course there are medications that can cure gout, fully removing the seed crystals. But as fate would have it, these drugs all cleared through the liver, so Lynda couldn't take them. The most potent pain killers also cleared through the liver, even were toxic to it, and the few painkillers she could take were of little help.

The only way to remove the inflammation left to us was a massive dose of steroids (prednisone) which was then slowly ramped down to avoid side effects. At least three times we rode the spike up, saw the gout clear, dropped slowly down to a dosage that her body could tolerate over time, only to see the gout flare up again.

Another drug, colchicine, was tried in place of the steroids, but that caused the worst hives Lynda had had since the laundry softener got her a week before our wedding.

Finally the docs hit on a 50/50 mixture of steroids and colchicine, the steroid just enough to keep away the hives while the colchicine kept away the gout.

It didn't take us long to find out why they tried to keep the steroid use to a minimum. It wasn't long after we got the gout under control that the steroids finally made themselves felt by getting to her sugar/insulin regulatory system and caused the onset of diabetes. We discovered this when she was so ill that we took her in to the ER and discovered a whopping blood sugar level of over 800. Normal blood sugar is just under 100; 200 is the point where chronic effects set in after awhile. 800 is considered immediately dangerous.

The most modern insulin control drugs (oral, long-acting) also clear through the liver, so we had to go the old fashioned injection route with 28 units twice daily.

The last pair of dominos were taken out by a triple whack of the encephalopathy, the wild blood sugar (causing dizziness and nausea) and her impaired walking and balance due to the gout. Lynda fell down the stairs—twice! The lesser one caused a sore coccyx and back muscle spasms. The worse one lead to ER room X-rays which revealed a cracked rib and a compression fracture of one vertebra—neither of which could be treated by anything more than mandatory bed rest. As if Lynda was going to go out and climb mountains, lift weights, or operate power machinery!

Perhaps it was a quadruple whack on those last dominos—the Zoloft she was taking to alleviate her anxious nightmares can also reduce caution in general, and may have made her overconfident on the stairs.

For all the pain and suffering of this period, the worst part was knowing that it would only get worse until her liver came, assuming it would come, and no way to know whether she'd be able to hold out that long—no way to know how long she'd have to hold out. Every time we thought we had things under control and her medications balanced out in a tolerable way, some other system of her body would go into play or give out.

They assured us that since the only thing fundamentally wrong was her liver, a transplant could result in total recovery. But could she take it that long? As she kept saying, over and over, "What next?"

9

Live Donor Prospects

	Winter	Spring	Summer	Fall
1988	(2) Engagement	(3) Wedding		
89-95	(4) Raising our Children			
1996			(5) Swelling	(1) Christmas
1997	(5) Diuretics	(5) Dehydrated	(5) Encephalop-athy	(5) Encephalop-athy
1998	(5) Encephalopa-thy	(5) Encephalopa-thy	(5) On the List	(6) Holding to Family
1999	(6) Holding to Family	(7) Big Crash, Shunt	(8) Dominos Falling	**(9) Live Donor?**
2000	**(9) Aborted Hopes**			

As Lynda waited for her transplant, we tried not to think much of where a liver would have to come from, and what it meant to hope it came soon. Your liver is a vital organ you can't do without, so a fully intact and functional liver can only come from someone who has no further use for theirs. And to make it seem all the more ghoulish, the donor must be freshly dead or legally dead (no brain function) with their body on life support.

One doctor wanted the best for Lynda, but was powerless to speed up the waiting process. He jokingly said the only thing he could do to speed things up was to go out and shoot five people—of the right blood type of course.

So there we were month after month waiting for someone to die under the proper circumstances, so that Lynda could get on about her own life. I'm sure it didn't bother me as much as it did Lynda—it was much more personal for her. You just have to adopt the attitude that people do die and it would be a shame to waste what they no longer need. But it does make you feel funny, hoping for a liver to come. What could you ask for in a prayer—beyond, "Thy Will Be Done"?

People are much more familiar with kidney transplants and hear stories about people donating a kidney to save somebody's life. Of course you have two kidneys and only one liver. Actually though, there is a way to do a live liver donation that makes sense.

It started by sharing a single adult donor's liver among several infants, but then a remarkable property of livers manifested itself. Normal livers are constantly renewing themselves—recall this is the capability that Lynda's liver had lost. Well, a portion of a liver transplanted into an infant still has that ability and so grows with the child. From there it is not too big a step to a live-donation of a portion of a liver to a baby and ultimately an adult donating *half* of their liver to another adult.

This was being done, on a very limited basis at this time. Both halves of the liver would grow back, and you'd end up, if all went well, with both adults having full livers—truly a miracle.

And so there in the wings hung the possibility of a live donation by someone willing to give up half of their liver for Lynda.

Of course such a donor is hard to come by. Besides being willing, they must have the same blood type (Rh doesn't matter) as well as being a physical match in size and shape as well as "plumbing" connections. In addition this person must be healthy and large—they really only move over 40% of the liver, so the donor must be bigger than the recipient—yet not too *thick* front to back so the liver *fits*.

Let me just say I'm glad I did not face the choice; I'm the wrong blood type. I'm not sure how I would have come out on the question—whether I would have felt willing to risk my children's last healthy parent in order to try and save the other. And this was because the grim fact was that there was a real chance—perhaps about 5% or even higher—that the donor would not survive. This was serious surgery and a serious risk to both people on the table.

For the longest time, as Lynda got sicker and sicker, no one stepped forward to be considered as a candidate donor. Lynda's family would not discuss it with her, and would not even tell their blood types.

Lynda was faced with dealing with the fact that no one in the entire world would risk their life to save hers. No one. Month after month, as she got worse, her nose was rubbed in this conspicuous lack. Now I won't deny that she was miserable, and unable to work or do anything meaningful during this period. But rationally I had to consider a few things without voicing them. Lynda could still wait her time in purgatory and get a liver in the end through normal channels. Her life was not in the balance yet, so we were weighing a quality of life issue (less than a year of virtual torture) vs. the risk of lost years of life by the donor. You would have to be very devoted to agree to that risk. The other thing was that if Lynda's condition worsened and it really did become a life-threatening situation for her, someone might still step forward. Then again, to be fair, Lynda's chances of surviving the surgery dwindled with her strength, so nothing was in clear black and white. People were dying waiting for livers.

Indeed, two people eventually did step forward as potential partial-liver donors.

The first was her childhood friend that Lynda considered a surrogate sister. Her "sister" had the right blood type and would do anything she could to help Lynda. However, her health was not good, and she didn't want Lynda's hopes to be raised until she knew for sure, for fear that those hopes would be dashed again.

This put me in an awkward position, seeing Lynda worried about getting a transplant, but, more, depressed by the feeling that she was alone and no one cared enough about her to even be tested. Ultimately I urged her sister to tell Lynda, and I think this helped, even though her sister was disqualified in the end. Her being overweight was theoretically fixable; with this to motivate her she might be able to solve a life-long weight problem. The final word though was her blood pressure—too high and no reasonable expectation of dealing with it.

The other person to step forward was quite a surprise. Recall that I wrote of Lynda's involvement with a friend who hosted many foster children, often infants, some with disabilities. The friend's older, biological children were of course very emotionally involved with these foster children, several of whom they ultimately adopted, and one son in particular must have been greatly impressed by Lynda's good work and personal qualities. It was one of her friend's sons, now a young man in his late twenties, who stepped forward to offer a portion of his liver.

Of course a great deal of testing was done before Lynda ever knew about the possibility. He was as healthy as a horse and, equally important; his vasculature was compatible with Lynda's. The testing included psychological exams, and the transplant center pulled no punches in explaining the dangers to the donor. At one point they said this might worse case estimate be as high as a 10% chance that he might not survive the experience, but he was not deterred. In truth he showed a great deal of curiosity and interest in the medical details.

The confidence of youth and their feeling of invincibility? Perhaps. More to the point was this family's strong Christian faith that God's Will Be Done. I wouldn't emphasize the flavor of their religion—some so-called Christians would consider this life-saving surgery an abomination and many would not risk their life for someone of a different faith. Rather we should focus on the strength of their faith and their belief in good works. These were simply Good People, you could tell that even without knowing that they had opened their hearts and home to so many needy children. I think they were particularly aware of all the vocal Christians in the area that talked up a storm but none the less would turn a blind eye to these needy innocents. Whereas, Lynda, a Jew, spent her life helping such children.

The last steps were a side-by-side eyeball comparison by the surgeons and a family meeting for us all to exchange views and set plans—a last chance to ask questions and for everyone to hear the same answers. This meeting was scheduled for January of 2000. What a way to start the New Year.

Our transplant center does get snow, but they were totally unprepared for the massive blizzard that hit, shutting down the entire region. Since we were facing our two families risking our lives by driving a nominal five hours through the Appalachians in the midst of this snow, which would double or triple the travel time if we made it at all, we of course postponed—'till February.

In February we got to meet the young man's fiancée at the family meeting, and she seemed proud and supportive. We set the date for the surgery to be the beginning of April, right after our family's annual Spring Break trip to Williamsburg Virginia with my parents, who would then stay on with the kids while I accompanied Lynda to the transplant center.

The week before we left, the very day my parents flew in from out West, the young man needed to talk with us. He was obviously torn up by the dilemma he faced. His fiancée was pregnant, he was getting married and had to face up to new responsibilities he hadn't had previously. For his own part he was still willing, but he could not put those risks onto a new wife and an unborn child. He had to back out of the surgery.

Lynda of course was devastated. I was a bit more retrospect in as much as I was still trying to understand what it took for someone to be willing to go to such sacrifice and risk in the first place. At the least, though, the timing was terrible.

I asked when the baby was due; the answer was November. This was nine months after our rescheduled trip to the transplant center. If the snow storm had not postponed the January meeting, we would have had no reason to delay the surgery for an upcoming trip, and Lynda might have had half this young man's liver inside her before anyone knew about the baby. Perhaps the baby might not have even been conceived.

As things turned out, this cancellation was actually not such a bad thing. After they opened Lynda up and discovered how rough her surgery and recovery were going to be, they told me that she might not have made it through with only half a liver to carry the load.

That freak snow-storm in January probably saved Lynda's life. Somebody surely was looking out for her.

10

The Call

	Winter	Spring	Summer	Fall
1988	(2) Engagement	(3) Wedding		
89-95	(4) Raising our Children			
1996			(5) Swelling	(1) Christmas
1997	(5) Diuretics	(5) Dehydrated	(5) Encephalopathy	(5) Encephalopathy
1998	(5) Encephalopathy	(5) Encephalopathy	(5) On the List	(6) Holding to Family
1999	(6) Holding to Family	(7) Big Crash, Shunt	(8) Dominos Falling	(9) Live Donor?
2000	(9) Aborted Hopes	**(10) Transplant**		

E-mail—Thursday, March 30, 2000.
Subject: Surgical Plan Change

Lynda's scheduled surgery is off. Complications in the life of the donor have closed down this option. We're back to waiting for the call to come the middle of the night—probably many months from now.

We are still going to Williamsburg for spring break, Friday 3/31 but I will be back in the office Monday, April 10th, for the duration.

Thanks for all the prayers,

-GERALD

Journal Entry—April 2nd, 2000

We had spent months working up to a Live Donor procedure, with our friend's son offering half of his liver. The Surgery was to be April 12, after our week in Williamsburg.

Wednesday the 29th we got the final word—he came to say his life had gotten too complicated, and he had new responsibilities now. The surgery was off. I went to the airport to pick up my parents and gave them the news.

Thursday I closed up shop at work—for a week now rather than two months. I sent e-mail notes saying the surgery was "probably months away". One friend at work came back saying surely not, perhaps days or weeks. I responded that I had spoken precisely and gave statistics to support that conclusion.

That night the call came—it wasn't even a whole day!

I was sitting on the floor in my PJ's packing for Williamsburg—consolidating my emergency bag with remnants from the last trip. This was sometime between 8:00 and 8:30. The caller was one of the liver coordinators—there was a liver—get in the car and come ASAP!!! We departed at 9:00 pm with everything I could think to grab and had an excited, keyed up but blessedly uneventful trip to the transplant center. We arrived at 1:45 am Friday morning.

We checked in at the ER just like any other patient, and slowly they got around to an IV and blood samples. Then later—almost as an after-thought—urine. Then another blood sample. They were supposed to get her 4:15 for 5:00 am surgery. Time went by…

Turns out Lynda had a new anti-body in her blood, probably due to the trans-fusions she got last summer. They had to get 20 units of blood products for this surgery, properly typed, and they had sent out the call to the Red Cross to find enough. If there were severe complications, they would have to give her less-than-perfectly compatible blood.

We went to a fifth floor room, and time dragged on—forms to fill out, etc. Finally they called us down to the holding room. Lynda went in with her "Jelly Music" (dreamy stuff from the Monterey Bay Aquarium Jellyfish exhibit) and pictures of the boys at 8:20 am. Five minutes later they brought the stuff back to me—she was asleep.

I went to the car, moved it, got established in the ICU waiting room. I was told it would be an hour hooking up tubes before they actually started. Appar-ently it was longer—I got word 10:20 or so that it had begun.

I fell asleep then, and got my only two hours of sleep. About noon Auntie arrived (well, sooner probably), and I was awakened by a phone call. About then, the doctors had an update for me.

Complication number one—as soon as they clamped off the portal vein that feeds the liver, her portal hypertension was the highest they had ever seen. It backed up fluid into her digestive track, and her intestines swelled up. Normally the size of one's finger, they became the size of my wrist. They couldn't get in to operate!

They rigged a bypass for the blood up to her neck/shoulder which took off the pressure and let them get to work, but visibility was poor. They warned me they expected leaks.

Complication number two—Lynda's liver was so badly scarred—so shrunken up and hard—that they had to "*burn*" it out piece by piece. I had the impression that it was adhered to things around it—between that and the limited visibility, her probability of bleeding would be higher. Some transplants the liver coming out looks not so bad—one piece and still flexible. Lynda basically didn't have any liver function left at all. I take it as a testament to how well we had fought to keep her balanced and functioning down to the point of surgery.

Saturday April Fool's Day was spent in a critical but not unusual state—kidney function low from the break in communication with the liver. No clotting factors yet from the new liver. A normal "seepage" effect from something like shock from the surgery.

In short, Lynda was leaking like a sieve, and they were pumping fluids through her at a phenomenal rate. There was a centrifuge unit like is used to donate platelets that was saving her red blood cells (actually not much was probably originally hers at that point), and they were giving them back to her.

Blood pressure was good—as long as they kept pumping her up—then it faded.

They expected this to last a day and then the clotting to kick in and start sealing up the leaks, letting the swelling go down.

Oh yeah, the swelling had been so bad that they couldn't close after the surgery—they had to put on a big plastic bandage to hold in her guts.

Anyway, this morning, the 2nd, Sunday, she was still losing fluid too fast—maybe even at an increased rate. So, they called us up at 7:00 am (new time, we sprang forward to daylight savings time) to get permission to go back in and clear out the old clots and such—which paradoxically keep her from clotting off where she needed it.

About 9:45 the surgeon came out to report progress—no obvious bleed points to repair—they added a few stitches here and there. I heard later that they removed *four liters* of clotted material.

She started a little urine—she needs a *lot* because that is how she'll get rid of the swelling ultimately—if she doesn't, they'll have to put her on a mini-dialysis machine.

We're back to waiting for the clotting to kick in, and the body to decide that it's okay, and seal up again (sort of like come out of shock). We need her veins to stop leaking fluid everywhere.

They can't let her wake up while her innards are still exposed—she swelled too much to close up again. Plan now is Monday (her birthday) they'll clean her up inside again. Maybe they will have to start the dialysis to get the swelling down.

Tuesday they'll either close her up the rest of the way, or put in a Gore-Tex layer (located more *inside* the abdominal wall this time) which may be semi-permanent enough to let her off the breathing tubes and wake up—this would be Tuesday at the earliest, as it all presumes she responds and pulls out of it.

This has been a hard surgery—ten hours the first time plus all these unexpected complications from the very high portal hypertension. Now the new liver is carrying quite a load with their dumping in clotting factor.

The surgeon says in retrospect she would not have been a good candidate for the live liver donor thing because half a liver would just not have been enough to carry the load. Good thing our friend's son backed out after all!!! Someone is really looking out for Lynda.

◆   ◆   ◆

11

Pumped Up and Pumping Down

	Winter	Spring	Summer	Fall
1988	(2) Engagement	(3) Wedding		
89-95	(4) Raising our Children			
1996			(5) Swelling	(1) Christmas
1997	(5) Diuretics	(5) Dehydrated	(5) Encephalopathy	(5) Encephalopathy
1998	(5) Encephalopathy	(5) Encephalopathy	(5) On the List	(6) Holding to Family
1999	(6) Holding to Family	(7) Big Crash, Shunt	(8) Dominos Falling	(9) Live Donor?
2000	(9) Aborted Hopes	(10) Transplant **(11) Closing Up**		

Journal Entry—Friday, April 7, 2000.

On Wednesday they did the partial close with a Gore-tex layer in place of natural tissue to hold everything in. They hope to close her the rest of the way next week.

Thursday she was starting to wake up a bit—enough to open her eyes (they were *very* yellow) but still not really showing signs of the liver doing its thing. Scan showed no bile leak.

Today she was a bit more awake—but still not up to complex things like choosing an audio tape. Her liver functions are finally all moving in the right direction, and she's breathing herself—with pressure assist from the machine. Got rid of the dialysis too—kidneys are okay. They hope to pull the breathing tube tomorrow. Lynda would feel much better if they did—or actually it's the other way around—they'd pull it if she felt better.

◆   ◆   ◆

Journal Entry—Sunday, April 9th, 2000.

We thought (again) we'd be pulling the tube today, but she has developed a touch of fever and infections (yeast and bacterial) in her urine and tra-chea—but not her abdomen. She's breathing very fast and shallow, so we're delaying the breathing tube pull. She's more alert, seemingly calm, but not able to track choices like which blanket to use—or have none at all.

◆   ◆   ◆

E-mail—Monday, April 10, 2000.
Subject: Lynda Update—10 days out

The major good news is the new liver is doing its job and the numbers get better every day.

The minor bad news is a host of little things that the surgeons feel they can easily deal with, but are delaying Lynda's recovery. She's still on a respirator, still not un-swollen enough to close up yet, still getting occasional dialysis until her kidneys "wake up" after the disruption, fighting some low-grade infections, still on enough sedatives to make her not care….about much of anything. Can't communicate. She will be a good while in the ICU still.

But, she is past the "acute" stage and has dodged several bullets. All those prayers are keeping her going. Many thanks.

-GERALD

Journal Entry—Wednesday, April 12th, 2000.

Still "tomorrow"—always tomorrow. They need to get fluid off to get the swelling down, to close her, to get the breathing tube out.

Today they started dialysis, and her blood pressure dropped to 85/40—alarming! So dialysis was cut short, couldn't take off a lot of fluid, and so the house that Jack wants to build is put off a bit more.

And the longer she is in ICU, the longer she's a target for some nasty infection to come along.

◆   ◆   ◆

E-mail—Friday, April 14th, 2000.

Subject: Lynda Status—Day 15

While progress is slow, I'm a little more upbeat about things after talking with the Doctor today.

They did a further partial closure today (25% more) and looked around. The fluid is gone and only the swelling of the liver itself is preventing a partial close (20% vs. 50% enlarged earlier). The liver functions are fine, and the swelling will come down with time. The mesh bandage they have in place would allow her to move out of ICU, for instance. They are happy with what they saw.

Lynda's kidney function is up and down, but progressing within the normal range for the difficulty of the surgery she had. They are confident it will return. Occasional dialysis will continue to supplement her kidney function—it is no longer required for fluid removal.

The VRE status (Vancomycin Resistant Enterococcus bacterium) was simply found colonizing her gut. She does *not* have an infection and Entrococcus is normally found in the gut—just not the Vancomycin resistant strains. If it were to get out of hand, there are other antibiotics that could be used, but at this time, all her cultures are showing up as negative for infections.

The next step is to get her off the breathing tube. The doc says patients progress at their own pace, with a whole bunch of snail-steps, then a big leap, then back to a snail's pace. No way to tell when her body will say "ready". To my eye her breathing was much stronger yesterday. This is really the only thing holding her in ICU at this time, and she could pop out of it any time.

Anyway, a bit more optimistic note than in the past. Thanks for all the prayers!

-GERALD

Journal Entry—Tuesday, April 18th, 2000.

Not much news. They did a 25% further close on Thursday—fluid was gone from intestines, but liver itself was still slightly inflamed—20% now vs. 50% earlier. It is getting better. The "squeeze" showed up as a slight set-back in her liver numbers, which otherwise show steady improvement.

Her kidneys are up and down, but the surgeon says she's following normal range for the difficulty of surgery she had. "She is no longer a statistical outlier" (i.e., her case no longer lay outside the normal range).

As of just before this surgery, she went "VRE" which means the natural entero-caucal bacteria in her gut has been colonized by a strain resistant to vancomycin, a popular and powerful antibiotic. Lynda does *not* have an infection (so I thought, I later learned that she did), and if she did get it there are other less effective antibiotics that would work. The VRE is a recognized problem, spreading through the hospital. To try to stem the spread they have special quarantine procedures now for Lynda—gowns and gloves. This wouldn't stop the kids from visiting (and they will be exposed at home), but this would make a visit more difficult. The post-surgical transplant apartments, where we expected to stay for a few weeks, would be better venue.

Last night her breathing was better—pressure support only. The tube pull is the next step. She can go to a regular room with the mesh on her abdomen and doing dialysis.

Last night her blood pressure was pretty low 85/24-> 85/22-> 80/12-> 78/25. I called this to the nurse's attention—they were short of staff and dealing with a crisis a few doors down. They said the dialysis took off too much fluid and fixed her up with IV's of albumen and fluid.

◆   ◆   ◆

Journal Entry—Wednesday, April 19th—Passover.

They finally sewed her up today. They mostly got the abdominal wall closed, with an area about the size of my hand in a permanent double gortex plus skin which will heal up just as strong as the rest.

Tomorrow they will pull the respirator—put a trachea tube if they have to.

◆   ◆   ◆

E-mail—Thursday, April 20, 2000.
Subject: Lynda Status—Day 21

Well, Lynda is still making slow progress forward. They managed to close her up yesterday (finally!). The breathing tube will come out tomorrow—50/50 chance they may have to put back in a (temporary, but more comfortable) trachea line. The liver continues to improve, but they are having to balance what fluid level is best for the liver vs. what is best for the kidneys. It will just take time to get it all to come together and "get well". At least another week in ICU—nobody willing to predict anything beyond that. Lynda has been just conscious enough to make facial expressions, but not really communicate. Here again she is gradually improving.

Thanks for all the prayers (and cards)!
-GERALD

Journal Entry—Friday, April 21ˢᵗ, 2000.

Auntie spelled me for the weekend, and I went home to see the boys. They were getting punchy, and it was Easter. Grandpa really thought they needed to see parents after three weeks.

While I was away they called for consent on some procedures. Seems Lynda had a bile-duct leak where the new liver was joined surgically. They had tried to come at it from below by going down the esophagus and up the bile duct, but the angle was bad, and they couldn't put in a tube-patch. So they tried coming through the skin and at it from above. They inserted a drain to get the bile away from the hole for four or five days to see whether it would seal itself up.

◆   ◆   ◆

Journal Entry—Monday, April 24ᵗʰ, 2000.

Auntie said that Lynda was awake but confused. Frankly I didn't think it was that bad when I got back. Of course I'd gotten used to seeing her encephalopathic.

They had also put in the trachea hole—easier to breathe and clean the mouth, but temporarily. Sure wish I could read lips. Lynda tries to say complex things, and won't confirm or give us feedback on my 20-question approach, so I'd say more "channeled" than confused.

◆   ◆   ◆

Journal Entry—April 25ᵗʰ, 2000

Rather more lucid and giving feed back. Definitely an "up" day.

◆   ◆   ◆

Journal Entry—Wednesday, April 26ᵗʰ, 2000.

She's very tired and getting worse by evening. Really hard to communicate, and she can't hold a thought long or give intelligent feedback. Also she has developed terrible shaking in the hands. I suspect build-up of encephalopathic waste products despite the 24-hour dialysis. Her kidneys aren't making any urine at all.

They deliberately are keeping fluid levels low via dialysis, because the liver needs it low to drain even though kidneys need it high to pee. Their experience is that if you get the liver working right, the kidneys will "wake up" and follow.

The 24-hour thing is more gentle on blood pressure—the big hit from regular hemo-dialysis on blood pressure is scary. This is much better than last week when I went in, and her blood pressure was very low (see the entry for 4/18). That was definitely the result of poor control trying to get fluid off—favoring the liver over the kidneys.

◆   ◆   ◆

12

Fighting to the Last

	Winter	Spring	Summer	Fall
1988	(2) Engagement	(3) Wedding		
89-95	(4) Raising our Children			
1996			(5) Swelling	(1) Christmas
1997	(5) Diuretics	(5) Dehydrated	(5) Encephalop-athy	(5) Encephalop-athy
1998	(5) Encephalopa-thy	(5) Encephalopa-thy	(5) On the List	(6) Holding to Family
1999	(6) Holding to Family	(7) Big Crash, Shunt	(8) Dominos Falling	(9) Live Donor?
2000	(9) Aborted Hopes	(10) Transplant (11) Closing Up **(12) Lingering**		

Journal Entry—Thursday, April 27th, 2000.

Talked with one of the resident physicians, new on the transplant team. Lynda is pooling fluid around the Gore-tex mesh. May be infected, may be blood. This *may* have been contributory to her state last night. They want to "clean her out" before it gets seriously infected, and she gets really sick.

They plan to replace this mesh with another sort that will dissolve away over time, leaving just scar tissue in her abdominal wall.

On another note, an old folkdance friend of ours from back home is in the hospital, operated on for a hole in her diaphragm which had been hanging around from a previous automobile accident. We sent get well flowers to her room—she's out of the ICU, and the surgery went well.

◆   ◆   ◆

Well, just talked to another resident regarding Lynda's surgery. They cleared out a fist-sized lump of puss, which had not really spread, so that was good. It was in the area of the bile leak, which could not now be located, so that was good. She said that they *did* find VRE inside her around the bile duct the last time she was opened up.

The liver was not so much *bleeding* as it was oozing from a large raw area in back. They are not real happy with the graft but hope that taking off the pressure will let it recover better.

They put a mesh in that dissolves away but did not close her. This resident seems to think it very likely that she'll have to be opened up again, but if not, the mesh will scar up, and she may some day need a skin graft over the area.

The surgeon said that she may some day need a new liver, but we don't have any figures on the likelihood of that. This was second-hand based on a comment he had made to the resident—he was not here to ask to make a guess.

E-mail—Thursday, April 27th, 2000.
Subject: Lynda Status—Day 28

Lynda is past the "acute phase" of this regime but has continued to have a few complications. Last weekend they rigged a drain to re-route her bile so a hole in her bile duct could self-seal. They got the tubes out of her mouth and put a temporary hole in her trachea to breathe—she is doing well with it and is completely off the ventilator, but she has no air flow to her vocal chords—wish I could read lips better! She is still getting dialysis because her kidneys haven't "woken up" yet.

Her alertness peaked about Tuesday, and she was her old self again, but has slowly lapsed back to confusion today. They've done a CT scan and found some bleeding on the back of her liver and fluid build-up around the gore-tex mesh. They are going to open her up again today to fix these problems, clean her out, and put in a different sort of mesh that dissolves away with time.

She was able to appreciate all the cards coming in—and the news of her big award at ETSU for long-term contribution to the Dept of Education.

Thanks for all the prayers and support—they continue to be needed!
-GERALD

◆   ◆   ◆

Journal Entry—Friday, April 28th, 2000.

She had very low mental function. Not even the bizarre Cheshire-cat smiles any more.

They were concerned that the liver may be squeezed too much and not getting enough blood, so they did an angio-gram, running fiber optic TV cameras down her arteries to see whether there were restrictions—she was okay.

◆   ◆   ◆

Journal Entry—Saturday, April 29th, 2000.

The Cheshire-cat smiles are back. The wound is not showing any sign of infection, but the liver biopsy showed mild regression; on a 9-point scale she was about a four where a healthy person is about a two. They just up the steroid for that. The first resident is concerned about the low mental state but can't put a finger on dominant cause—"multi-factor—inoperable".

They will move her to a bigger room with more light today—that may help any "psychotic" component of her mental status. "You'd be surprised" the nurse says.

◆   ◆   ◆

E-mail—Sunday, April 30th, 2000.
Subject: Lynda Status—Day 31

Lynda has been fighting some infections and fever the last few days. They bumped up her steroids to counteract the very mild beginnings of rejection. After being pretty alert on Tuesday, she has slid downhill and was pretty much asleep all this morning. She is back on the ventilator, and they will probably sedate her the rest of today to slow down her breathing rate. Her kidneys are still pretty much shut down, and she's getting dialysis, though everybody says that kidneys usually rebound from this state. Tests show her liver is getting the blood flow it needs. All we can do for her is wait, and pray.

Thanks for all the prayers,
-GERALD

Journal Entry—Monday, May 1st, 2000.

The second resident called this morning saying mixed things. They were puzzled by her fever, which was down some. They saw fluid in her lungs with X-ray and went in to suck a sample out to culture. Inside she didn't really *look* like she had pneumonia, but the lab work would take time. Now X-rays show less fluid—perhaps because they sucked it out!

In doing this procedure, they caused some bleeding and had to give Lynda more blood and platelets—she is not clotting well. I noticed some serious bruises developing on her hands around old IV sites.

Lynda is reported to be pretty much unconscious today—grimaces easily when touched—sedated, so that her breathing will be more normal. She's up to breathing to the rhythm of the ventilator again.

Also the "open" chest mesh is bleeding some (as expected?) hence the need for blood.

◆ ◆ ◆

Journal Entry—Tuesday, May 2nd, 2000.

Called me for consent to change dialysis catheter site from neck to groin/leg. Apparently site showed infection when they "changed plastic".

She's still zonked today.

Last night was still awake after 1:00 am when an old man was calling for help in the hallway at the transplant hotel/suites. He was asking for somebody to call the police and saying someone was keeping him away from proper medical care. By time I was in the hall in only trousers, two hotel employees were escorting him toward the front desk, asking why they should call the police.

[Turns out the man was waiting for a liver transplant—went violently delusional in the ICU for several days—was sedated—then passed away. Later, I met the family at the family housing.]

Earlier this week my doorknob broke (green light when I ran the card but no mechanical action), and they took a couple hours to disassemble the knob and get in. I slept that night with "safety chain" only, and they fixed it in the morning (I didn't want to move all my junk to another room). [This happened again later when our old folk-dance friend was staying in the family housing to visit Lynda.] Something about me and doors in this place—about three times my key card expired while I was off doing laundry, and last summer the Caravan door all but fell off, and I had to get it welded back on by a local mechanic.

◆ ◆ ◆

E-Mail—Friday, May 5th, 2000.
Subject: Lynda Status—Day 36

Lynda is coming off a 10-day period of fighting infections and is back on the mend, with no fever or other such signs. She is trying to talk but doesn't make much sense—of course that is 90% my poor lip-reading skills. She's still on a ventilator, but she's initiating her own breaths again. The pressure support required is being turned down each day. She's still on dialysis. I am going home to spend my birthday weekend with the boys—Lynda's sister will be here with her during this time.

Take care all,

-GERALD

Journal Entry—Wednesday, May 10th, 2000.

Yesterday Lynda developed a 100.6°F fever, and her blood pressure did not "bounce back" when they finally dried her out—the latter being the desirable end result of a month of dialysis.

The hope is that this was the necessary condition for her liver to start working.

They got consent to do three things; CT scan, put a swan catheter in her heart to monitor blood pressure/fluid issues, and another broncho-scope to check out "patches" seen in her lung X-ray.

Results: Her lungs look good—pending results of cultures. The noisy fluid is really all in her trachea area because she's too weak to cough enough to keep it clear.

The swan catheter confirmed her fluid level was good—vessels were vaso-dilated which is consistent with an infection.

CT scan sees a pocket of fluid that has formed up behind her liver.

Today, gave consent to Radiology to go in with needles to drain the fluid (not clear now if they were going to leave in a drain), and of course culture it.

A third resident (or intern, hard to tell the difference) yesterday said Lynda isn't moving because she is so *weak*—that the nurses say she does move *some*. Lynda's surrogate "sister" who is a therapist disagrees—that all the motion is spastic, and that Lynda is hallucinating constantly. Time will tell about the ulti-mate outcome. Quality of life issues need to be considered. My feeling is that is not my call as long as there is reasonable hope of Lynda being aware enough to make her own decisions. My only call is on the topic of her prospects of recover-ing mental function—which of course the doctors don't say is really any question at all. Lynda is still in the typical range of recovery time, though moving to the slow end of the range. But then if you think about it, Lynda's new liver has not been to optimal fluid-recovery status until the last couple days, so in one sense, this "month" doesn't really "count" as recovery time.

Hmmm, yesterday the nurse mentioned that Lynda was getting a *little bit* of Dopamine—which I now recall is used to keep blood pressure up. Last summer she was on dopamine when they watched for heart arrhythmia—which happened.

◆   ◆   ◆

Journal Entry—Saturday, May 13th, 2000.

What they found in response to the blood pressure problem was that she *did* have some pneumonia, and they drained the fluid found in her abdomen. It ultimately did *not* culture out positive, but Lynda did rally after this. When I got back on Thursday (from visiting back home on my birthday), she was alert and expressive. Not up to 20 questions but definitely appropriate facial expressions.

Friday did not look as good. Today she is completely unresponsive, and her eyes only cracked open.

The surgeon described what they are doing regarding contingencies, while giving the current medicines time to work.

—Searching for other infection sites.

—Boosting adrenaline/changing to a natural adrenaline to get her blood pressure in line (that will not suppress immune system as much).

—Eliminating immune suppressants—probably take a week to develop rejection problems. She is *not* healing, though her white count is going up, and liver numbers are actually getting better.

They are holding off on more CT scans, and opening her up to rummage around for infection sites is definitely something they will leave for a later resort.

The nurses and the doctor keep saying that they've seen people sicker than this recover, but they're not putting it in high-probability terms either.

I find I can't do more than drain her respiratory lines (which accumulate fluid despite the traps) and get rid of pressure points on her body due to position, and give her a good suction around the mouth then head out. It is just too emotionally exhausting to stay by her side.

◆   ◆   ◆

13

Beacon in the Darkness

	Winter	Spring	Summer	Fall
1988	(2) Engagement	(3) Wedding		
1989	**(13) Reflections on Adoption**			(4) Adoption
90-95	(4) Raising our Children			
1996			(5) Swelling	(1) Christmas
1997	(5) Diuretics	(5) Dehydrated	(5) Encephalop-athy	(5) Encephalop-athy
1998	(5) Encephalopa-thy	(5) Encephalopa-thy	(5) On the List	(6) Holding to Family
1999	(6) Holding to Family	(7) Big Crash, Shunt	(8) Dominos Falling	(9) Live Donor?
2000	(9) Aborted Hopes	(10) Transplant (11) Closing Up (12) Lingering	**(13) Beacon**	

So there I was, caught in an intolerable box, between staying and caring for Lynda, my physical inability to keep up the contact, the grumblings from home that the boys were starting to get restless and needed their Dad, and worst of all, the very real and likely prospect of losing Lynda permanently.

In hind sight, what I had to do may have been obvious, but at the time, the very conflict that was burning me up with fatigue was blocking my ability to deal with it all.

All I knew was that the situation was intolerable, so I listened to my body and withdrew for a time to sort it all out. My day to day moral yardstick was failing me, and I needed to reassess my basic values. I needed to find a beacon for my life that would help me find my way.

Fortunately, my life choices had given me some experience with this. Lynda and I had had to sort out our values together in starting our family, particularly because of the way we did it. That "thinking about what I valued in my life" helped me to again find my way.

Lynda and I had waited most of a year after getting married before trying to have children. We figured we owed it to the children to be sure we were sufficiently compatible to stay together long enough to raise them. Also, we were aware that we wouldn't have much time for each other once the kids came along. We agreed that a year would be a good amount of time, but some of the time of a pregnancy might count towards that, as well as time we had together before we were married. So by late in 1988 we had put away the birth control, and were trying for a child.

The results were a real anticlimax. We may as well have not worried about birth control the first part of our marriage because it made no difference. Granted, Lynda missed a few periods but nothing ever lasted long enough for a viable pregnancy to become established naturally. She never even got far enough along to call it a miscarriage. Problems at this early stage can be with the mother's hormone system, or it could be genetic with either partner contributing non-viable DNA code that produces a pre-fetal cluster of cells that does not grow properly and the mother's body does not recognize as viable, instead aborting it early on. I imagine there are many other possible reasons for why we were not fertile, *together*. It seemed to be a pretty clear fact, whatever the cause.

When we realized that we had fertility problems, Lynda informed me of two things. One was what a horror it would be for her to undergo fertility treatments (and expensive), not to mention uncertain and full of heartbreak, but that she'd do it if I absolutely insisted. The other was that there were a lot of people who adopted children, and that she had thought about it a lot and was comfortable with adoption.

The tales of what it would take to create a baby inside Lynda were pretty scary, especially since we did not know what our problem was. We could be throwing away money in the 5-digit range every time we tried something, which amounts to a very expensive lottery ticket indeed! The indignity of what Lynda would have to suffer, the potential dangers and side effects, and the roller-coaster ride of uncertainty were, to say the least, not very attractive. And how could I ask Lynda to shoulder that load so that I could follow the "traditional" expectations of a father? I mean, biology has tipped the workload of childbirth heavily against the mother. We men make up for it in part by taking the heavy jobs by tradition and dying an average of 4 years earlier due to stress, health, and accidents. But could I ask Lynda, who started out with a fear of doctors, to tilt the balance even further? This is the lady whose blood pressure goes through the roof when she just steps into a doctor's office? This is the lady who had never been hospitalized in her life? (I had behind me the experience of having tonsils and wisdom teeth out, as well as having spent the first several years of my life with ophthalmologists, and had eye surgery twice before I can even remember).

Add in Lynda's age, and what the extra dangers were to both the mother and the child for having a first pregnancy after the age of 40. We could be responsible for trying very hard to bring a damaged baby into the world. In Lynda's work she had seen a lot of damaged babies, and knew what that meant.

Finally, consider the fact that Lynda had a career that she intended to pursue, a career with far more social relevance and impact on society than my own. Sure, I earned more money than she did, but what were my chances of changing the world with a new and better plastic? I would have to be asking her to sacrifice career to undergo these horrible procedures in order to sacrifice even more career to bear the baby.

I had already faced the ghost of non-traditional parenting role models when accepting the idea of a working mom. I was fine with sharing the childcare, sharing the housekeeping. I enjoyed kids and had been doing quite well by myself, domestically speaking, for a half-dozen years thank-you-very-much. Was I now going to turn my back on that accord and expect her to go to the opposite extreme? The intellectual, rational answer was quite clear; I should accept the concept of adoption. But, it felt like I was being asked to sacrifice something in order to make our relationship work.

And what a sacrifice!

All my expectations would have to change, of course. Gone was the traditional view of nursing a wife with "cravings" and being gallant to her for the baby's sake. Gone was the rush to the hospital and the pacing in the waiting room. Gone were the games of whose nose the baby had, whose eyes, whose chin. I was being asked to accept a baby who didn't look like me, and might be very different from me in ways I didn't know yet.

Of course I had never discussed this sort of thing with my parents, and so I had a sense of wanting to make them proud by giving them grandchildren, again in the traditional way. How would they feel about my going off and doing something different? Our family had a lot of special talents—very high IQ's for the whole bunch—and had a bit of an elitist streak, that our family was better than everybody else (face it, whose family doesn't?)

Society is full of examples of men obsessed with their wife's fidelity and needing to know who fathered their child. An "unfaithful" wife, who was responsible for the situation, was still jealously guarded as their possession in a macho world, whereas the question of parentage determined whether the baby was "theirs" and whether they had a social obligation to raise them. This sort of thing gave legal grounds for divorce. It took a special kind of nobility for a man to turn a blind eye to questions of parentage, and raise a child in that situation as his own. Of course this was, in a sense, accepting something after the fact—I was considering doing this on purpose. These were the role models given to me by society as an American Male.

Again, I felt like I was being asked to sacrifice in order to do the "right thing". Lynda would have stood aside if I wanted to marry someone else that would be able to give me children the usual way, she said. As if I was going to say, "Fine Honey, let's put everything on hold awhile while I rethink whether I want to be with you." That would work, sure! Again, my sense of responsibility would not let me do any such thing—feeling like I was trapped wouldn't get me anywhere. I was in this situation because I chose to stay there. I would just have to reconcile my feelings with my head. It was something I felt some pride in being able to do. I needed to analyze my feelings.

So I faced the great debate—Nature or Nurture. Anybody who knows dog breeds knows there is a lot on the nature side; the temperaments of a Chihuahua, vs. that of a Golden Retriever, are quite different and reproducible. On the other hand everyone will agree that a bad environment—poor nourishment, disease, and neglect—can have a terribly adverse impact. Academic studies comparing factors in twin studies and the like tend to come up with the compromise 50/50 relationship position, but how did they choose their measures? This just means they chose a balanced set of parameters to measure; I might not agree on what it is that makes me *ME*.

Let's look at family. All of us kids had higher IQ's than our parents—there is a good argument for nurture. I think my mom did a particularly good job with us; she had a bachelor's degree in biology and spent a lot of time on her grand-mother's farm, so I'm sure she did very well for us. (And my Dad knocked him-self out providing for us. We were not rich, but we had everything we needed as kids.)

Our cousins were a mixed bag, ranging from English Boarding School to cut-ting grass for a living. We weren't exactly city folks, but many of our cousins were definitely rural, and we kids thought some of them were kind of slow in many ways.

On the other side, we have examples of charity and good works ranging from church to Scouts (my mom lead Scouts, taught leaders, and went on to set up classes for leader training). Much glory and nobility goes to the credit of those who work for the good of all humanity. Wars are fought brother vs. brother over politics and religion. Clearly there are some things that society places ahead of family, even if the old saying goes, "Blood is thicker than water". You could argue, and therefore one has to decide for oneself what things are important to each of us.

Let's talk genes. We share something like 99% of our genes with chimpanzees. Of course you could argue that that 1% is pretty darned important. But how does the human-chimp relationship compare to the Chihuahua-Golden Retriever analogy? How much of what we care about is derived from that 1% of our genes?

Racial groups is where most people take this, but that's too simplistic. The world comes to a lot of grief in friction supposedly over racial differences, but really those fights are about cultural differences and political/religious differences—things too hard for one to assess on first encounter. So, as a psychological short-cut, people fixate on what they can see—which usually means skin color. What self-delusion to think that one glance can tell it all! Australian aborigines, for instance, are dark because they are adapted to hot climates just like central Africans—they share little else except that both are examples of local variants on Homo Sapiens. Every race has such relatively minor adaptations. Within a race you have a broad range of much more important things, harder to come by like intelligence, strength, endurance, resistance to disease. Should charm and beauty be on this list? Is there a gene for leadership and honor, or for good character? The natural selection of our genes to whatever extent it continues on, does so on a much more complex field than just black and white.

So if I want to be a father, and pass my genes on to future generations, it's time for an "up close and personal" genetic audit.

I have very pale white skin. In many societies this is considered a status symbol because the ruling classes are descended from pale invaders who brought guns and, more lethal, small pox, to conquer those that came before. To me, pale skin means I sunburn in a heartbeat. My ancestors were adapted to cold climates, and I'm good in frostbite territory, but I'm miserable in heat and humidity. I'm subject to untold rashes and fungi because my body must sweat to stay cool, most places. I think I'll vote "Nay" on passing on any extreme of local climate adaptation!

Another thing my ancestors brought—some were Irish immigrants escaping from the potato blight. There are anecdotes that prove to my own satisfaction that those with a good sense of color could cope with a blighted potato, but those who could not ate them and got sick. As a result of this selection factor, a high proportion of folks descended from Irish immigrants are color blind—not me but my Grandfather, and I might be a carrier.

Another thing that runs in the family, is a relatively long spine and short legs—a wrestler's build I'm told. I suppose there is some psychological value to sitting tall at a conference table. I must note, however, that a high proportion of my relatives have back trouble—including me. This is another one my descendants can do without.

Allergies run in my family—though some would debate how much of that comes from ones genetic component. It can be miserable—though it may provide more protection in an environment beset by microscopic insults. A curious advantage it confers is the opposite of "dry mouth syndrome"—the constant fluid bath on my teeth meant no cavities until I was an adult. Bottom line, the jury is still out on the ideal immune system function—I certainly have no basis for wanting to pass on my own particular combination.

My wisdom teeth grew in at an angle—if I'd had few other teeth left by my teens like the cave men, these might have pushed my remaining teeth to the front where they were more useful. To me, though, it meant a painful oral surgery in my teenage years.

Let's not even talk about huge arches and triple wide feet.

The kicker though is my eyes. I manifest a recessive gene that popped up in several male ancestors and a couple cousins—we have strabismus, or crossed eyes. Two surgeries as an infant may have corrected the gross anatomy, but my brain never learned to fuse the twin images it received. I thus have no depth perception. It's very hard to find a positive side to this disability, but I'll give a shot for the record. Many academic studies have linked physical disabilities, particularly bad eyes, with mathematical aptitude. So the argument runs that the brain-power freed up by not having to fuse 3-D images instead contributed to an obscenely high IQ and/or mathematical ability.

There perhaps is where the rubber meets the road on a personal assessment of my position in Darwin's game of life. Proposition: I should have children to further a race of googly-eyed super-geniuses that will some day rule the world. Reminds me of "Dr. Who and the Daleks"—these monstrous blobs of brain protein encased in a heartless mechanical life support system.

Let's get real folks—there is nothing special in my genes that I'd like to keep and that is significantly different from that of the other 6 billion examples of Homo Sapiens currently expressed on this planet.

Yes, I'm particular to my own brown eyes and red-blond-brown hair that sparkles like the stone called tiger's eye. But then I find Polynesians look very attractive as well. I used to kid my little sister, who had blue eyes, telling her the Native

American's point of view who, upon encountering the English, thought that their heads were hollow, and you could see the blue sky behind, shining through.

Let's just say that never in my life have I relied on my genes as a source of pride. My pride and self-esteem came from my mind and what I did with it. As my mother would say as she clucked her tongue over and A *minus*, it's not how smart you *are* but what you do with it.

And that is the basis of every war of culture, religion, political difference, of ideology and values. The world is a battle ground of *values*, more intense now than genetic selection ever was. (Footnote: If this wasn't clear when I wrote it, the subsequent events of September 11, 2001 certainly made this point clear!)

I got a chuckle out of one example of culture vs. genes. When I came to the Appalachians from California, and other points west, I physically blended right in with the Scotch-Irish that dominated the area, and yet I had such trouble understanding the local accent that I was helpless trying to understand a high school girl trying to take my fast food order at KFC, who turned "original or crispy" into three syllables. On the other hand, there were many college educated people who, like myself, came into the area for jobs. One such was the social worker I met when I volunteered at Big Brothers, who was from Kansas and spoke like I did—and she was black. I got a chuckle out of the fact that I felt more kinship for her than I did for the white folk I encountered on the street.

So what is it about myself that I do find special, uniquely me, and worthy of self-loyalty? We were always told that we had very high IQ's, but that just meant more was expected of us. Being intelligent was not a state of grace, it was a talent that would be a shame to waste. Your choices and your efforts are what counts. Or, to put it in the electronics age—it's the software, not the hardware, which matters. *Values* count.

So how does that apply to adopting children? If I want to pass on what is truly "me and mine", then the hardware was the least important thing. What mattered is the values you held, and lived by, and passed on to your children.

It didn't matter where the genes came from, what mattered was that you took the responsibility to care for them, to teach them the best you knew how, love them, and be a hero for them to look up to—to aspire to be like.

And so I came around to Lynda's point of view, wise woman that she was, and embraced adoption. Let me tell you that when they place an infant in your arms, and tell you the baby is yours, and that you are responsible—all the doubts about adoption vanish.

This was why Lynda and I came together—to form a family, to dedicate our lives to raising these boys the best we knew how.

And so with Lynda's body failing her, I knew where my responsibility lay, to the boys and the vision of hope for *them*, which I shared with Lynda. I had tried my best to bring these boys' Mama home for them, but the medical aspects were beyond me now. I was doing no more good at the transplant center.

I was needed at home—that's where I belonged. Whether Lynda ultimately lived or not, I wanted to be able to say I did my best to keep her vision alive.

And so our joint dream, a vision of a family that we had together, became my beacon. By this standard I could judge the right thing to do. I would do what I could for Lynda's body—little enough now—but I would do everything to keep the boys from taking too much harm from this situation. I would make life as normal for them as possible. I belonged home with them.

I took this a step further—what would I do if Lynda passed on? I couldn't resume a life of care-free bachelorhood. My obligations were clear—I had to find these boys another mother, and not just any stranger. These boys were already coping with growing up adopted, which meant realizing, typically as teens, that if *one* family gave them up once, why should *this* family be any different? These are some basic levels of insecurity that they would have to deal with already—then throw on top losing their mother. I needed to have a plan ready so that I could tell them what to expect even as I broke the news about their mother, if and when.

Who on Earth could step into those shoes in a natural way? Only one person at that time—"Auntie", the boys' godmother, an old college chum of Lynda's who was already a part of the boys lives—if somewhat geographically distant.

I wrote a long letter to Auntie explaining the situation and my fears. I felt pretty close to her, as she had been calling daily for updates about Lynda, and had even spelled me occasionally in my vigil. I asked her not to answer now, but to be aware that if Lynda died, time would be of the essence for protecting those boys' fragile psyches. I would be asking her whether she would come join me to raise them—that I would welcome her on whatever terms she chose regarding the relationship between us, but for the sake of the kids she must be prepared to answer yes or no on a moment's notice.

With a mission in my heart and a plan in my head, I knew my way for the first time in weeks, and headed home with determination.

14

Long Distance Support

	Winter	Spring	Summer	Fall
1988	(2) Engagement	(3) Wedding		
1989	(13) Reflections on Adoption			(4) Adoption
90-95	(4) Raising our Children			
1996			(5) Swelling	(1) Christmas
1997	(5) Diuretics	(5) Dehydrated	(5) Encephalop-athy	(5) Encephalop-athy
1998	(5) Encephalopa-thy	(5) Encephalopa-thy	(5) On the List	(6) Holding to Family
1999	(6) Holding to Family	(7) Big Crash, Shunt	(8) Dominos Falling	(9) Live Donor?
2000	(9) Aborted Hopes	(10) Transplant (11) Closing Up (12) Lingering	(13) Beacon **(14) Long Dis-tance**	**(14) Rehab**

E-mail—Monday, May 15th, 2000.
Subject: Lynda Status—Day 46

Lynda continues to fight infections and is only marginally conscious, part of the time. They have had to resort to tricks like stopping her immune suppression medicine to give her a better chance to fight back, knowing that they can only do this for about a week before rejection symptoms start to crop up. Definitely into second-tier type strategies but not into the desperate ones yet.

Her condition has been up and down on a daily basis for awhile—currently they seem to have a leg up and are able to reduce blood-pressure boosting medications which were needed to offset the effects of the infection (pneumonia mainly). She is still on ventilator and continuous dialysis to control fluid levels, but is resting better. Obviously the body only can keep fighting so long.

The doctors and nurses all say they have seen sicker people recover (but that's different from saying that most such people do). They tell me not to give up hope

yet, so keep those prayers coming—they are as much needed as ever. Thanks for all the support.
    -GERALD

E-mail—Wednesday, May 17th, 2000.
Subject: Lynda Status—Day 48
    Lynda has had an "up" day—her lips are moving a mile a minute, and she is showing a full range of emotional facial expressions. She still thinks we're stupid for not understanding her and won't play "20 questions" to communicate. The ventilator is all the way down. We'll be trying to get her off it and talking with a valve device in the next couple days.
    At the same time they keep finding and reacting to possible infection sites—2 in the last two days. She's going to get another abdominal drain to take care of one of them. Her condition is "fragile", and the rally came largely because they turned down her immune suppressants temporarily. They're giving her dopamine so they can keep pumping off fluid in an effort to get her liver functions where they need to be.
    Keep the faith,
    -GERALD

Journal Entry—Thursday, May 18th, 2000

Lynda has been responding to the treatments and is better each day. Today she is able to answer a couple questions and is very animated. They're only leaving her on dopamine so they can keep doing dialysis. They're doing a bladder flush due to infection and put in a new drain for abdominal fluid (not certain-maybe decided on the fly to replace old instead of put in new). She's still positive for pneumonia and of course can't stay off the immune suppressants forever.
    They're talking about removing the ventilator completely soon—too late for today though.

◆   ◆   ◆

Journal Entry—Monday, May 22nd, 2000.

We had some uncertainty over the weekend. Lynda had some stomach pain (X-rays showed nothing) and was loopy and sleepy from the painkiller. A friend from work saw her bright Friday afternoon then pained Friday night. Lynda slept a lot the rest of the time she was here. I asked her afterwards whether she was extra tired or just that being with her friend made her feel better—I distinctly saw her lips sync, "I felt better". Will have to tell the friend.

Today she is scheduled for a trachea valve so she can talk. This week they hope to get her up in chairs. Things are generally looking up, but she's still very sick, fragile, and is bleeding many places including lungs.

One point I learned—the body usually only fights one thing at a time, so the chances of rejection while she's fighting pneumonia are reduced. Even so, the threat of infection is worse, and they can tolerate a little bit of rejection symptoms if they had to. The trick is starting up the Prograf (immune suppressant) again when she "gets better".

◆   ◆   ◆

E-mail—Monday, May 22, 2000.
Subject: Lynda Status—Day 53

Lynda is doing about the same. A good old mundane digestive tummy ache (she has been being tube fed) caused her some pain, so the painkillers have put her on cloud 9 off and on the last few days. She's more comfortable than previously, but one has to worry whether she's getting better fast enough before something else comes along (she is still fighting junk in the lungs). They're talking about putting in a valve so she can talk this week, and trying to get her up sitting in a chair. She's off the ventilator about 80% of the time and breathing fine with just oxygen enrichment.

Keep up the prayers.
-GERALD

Journal Entry—May 24th, 2000.

Yesterday I had an appointment to discuss Lynda's prognosis with the doctors. Many people worried that Lynda might just hang on for a year bouncing from one infection to the next in misery with no real chance of recovery.

I learned that they really have a systematic review—they would tell me if there was something broken that can't be fixed—and there is not. Actually with liver transplants, nothing is really bad except the liver and with that replaced, either they get steadily better, or you've got a catastrophic failure. The liver really is the central metabolic organ and the barometer of how the body is doing. I asked if Lynda might be "stuck" in this state indefinitely, but they assured me she couldn't stay both stable and low functioning for months on end like a stroke victim could. She would either get better, or much worse. The danger is that an infection could get out of control and kill her fast—she could die in 2 days. But the strong undercurrent is the liver getting better.

In fact Lynda is rallying—she is scooting around in the bed and quite lucid. Agreed with the need for me to go back and be with the boys!

I gave her the ruby slippers music box finally. "There's No Place like Home!", and she can still make it if she just keeps dodging the infection long enough.

◆　　◆　　◆

Journal Entry—Wednesday, May 31st, 2000.

The two month anniversary of the surgery and Lynda is doing great. They're keeping the ventilator on nights to get good deep breaths, but during the day they let her have the valve to talk.

Turns out she didn't remember anything before today. They said to expect "ICU psychosis" until she got out to a quieter, regular room. She had dream compulsions to talk to some doctor from Sri Lanka and didn't believe me or the nurse that she had a new liver. She thought she had a couple days to live, and that we were so mean to lie to her about such an important thing.

Then, later, one doctor came by and told her the same thing—she had a new liver—and she was soooo happy—manic—thanking everyone and bouncing out of her skin. Eventually she asked for painkiller and slept like a log all night.

Quite a contrast—earlier she was saying the hospital was not a safe place—people came in and did things to her, and she wondered whether it would be safer sleeping in the car. She tried a dozen different ways to convince me to help her get up out of her chair and go—with a strong element of hunger and needing food. She wouldn't believe she couldn't go because of all the IV's including dialysis lines and was just plain mad.

◆　　◆　　◆

Journal Entry—Thursday, June 1st, 2000.

She's still sleeping like a log!!! Finally able to get some rest. I sat and watched her sleep for one to two hours.

◆　　◆　　◆

E-mail—Friday, June 2nd, 2000.
Subject: Lynda Status—Day 64

Lynda is actually doing pretty well. She seems to be responding to treatments for her infections/pneumonia. She is no longer coughing up blood, is off the ventilator except at night. She is actually awake and has a valve in her trachea tube so that she can talk. Not surprisingly she is quite confused about her situation and doesn't understand why she can't just get up and walk out. She passed the swallowing test and has started back on food—clear liquids & jell-o.

She is still on dialysis, though her kidneys have put out a few cc's of urine, and we expect her to follow the norm (for a change) and have her kidneys wake up. In the meantime, her blood pressure is still on the low side which is limiting how aggressive they can be with the dialysis. Her liver numbers are about 2.5 (down from 10) where normal is in the 1-2 range, so that is going very well.

Lynda will be some time recovering her strength. In the mean time I am going back to home to work and take care of the boys. Various friends will visit Lynda during this less dramatic time. I will need to go back when she is closer to discharge—which may only be a few weeks if things continue to go well.

Thanks for all the support,

-GERALD

E-mail—Thursday, June 8, 2000.
Subject: Lynda Status—Day 70

Good news! Day 70 of Lynda's stay at the transplant center, and she is finally being transferred out of Intensive Care! This means she is stable enough not to require constant life-support (ventilator etc.)—a major mile stone! She is going today to a "Critical Care Step-Down Unit" which will still not allow allergens (no flowers). I'm not sure whether she'll have access to a telephone, though speaking with the valve on her Trachea Tube may make comprehensible phone conversations impractical anyway—time will tell.

Lynda is still weak as a kitten and needs her kidneys to "wake up" to get off dialysis, so she is still weeks away from full discharge. But hey! This is progress!

-GERALD

E-mail—Friday, June 16ᵗʰ, 2000.
Subject: Lynda Status—Day 78

Lynda continues to make baby steps forward. Her pneumonia seems to be clearing up, and the fluid pooling in her abdomen (leaky spots from surgery) while not gone is minor enough not to be a cause for concern. Her liver enzyme levels are "twitching" around a bit. They think means she's done fighting infections. They also need to start her back on the full immune suppression medication. Medically she seems to be past all the life-threatening stuff (hence out of the ICU), but she has a lot of recovering to do:

- Kidneys—still "asleep" but they said it would take several weeks. Several hours dialysis every day or two.

- Bile Duct—still a leak but they hope it will close up without further intervention as she gets stronger & better nutrition. Bile draining through a tube in her side.

- Eating—a few bites then dry heaves later. Still a feeding tube up her nose.

- Strength—not able to stand yet, but getting PT and doing better. Can form letters like kindergartener.

- Confusion—very interactive but grip on reality fades in and out. Asks not to be left alone. Asks for impossible things.

- Breathing—in through the valved trachea tube, out through the mouth, talks like Minnie Mouse with a head cold.

- Hearing—seriously impaired—they are doing tests today to see whether it is permanent or just fluid buildup.

Discussed when it would be appropriate to have the kids visit her. She may or may not be a heart-warming sight (as opposed to scary) by 4th of July weekend. They couldn't offer odds on whether she would be out to a regular room (vs. step-down where she is now) by then.

Keep up the prayers—many thanks!

-GERALD

Journal Entry—June 19th, 2000.

Lynda's doing much better—getting smaller trachea tube, going back on some immune suppressants, peed some (still unbalanced electrolytes), so kidneys are starting to wake up. Still problems with the leaky, and possibly infected, bile duct and also piss poor hearing. We tried to talk on the phone, but I couldn't convince her I wasn't our son!

◆   ◆   ◆

E-mail—Monday, June 19th, 2000.
Subject: Lynda Status—Day 81

Good news! Lynda has moved to a regular room! Thus the ban on allergens (flowers) is lifted…While there is a phone in the room, she is not yet able to use it herself (hearing & mobility problems). Room number is 5232, but if she moves any more that may or may not be helpful. Lynda continues to make baby steps forward (figuratively)—her kidneys are producing fluid, though not yet balancing electrolytes.

The long-range plan has changed—rather than being discharged to an apartment near the transplant center, Lynda is likely to go to a rehabilitation center in the tri-cities area to build back her strength. This is still some weeks away—I hope to visit with the boys over 4th of July weekend.

-GERALD

E-mail—Wednesday, June 21, 2000.
Subject: Lynda—Woops!

I was in error about flowers. For some reason they are still not allowed—sorry for the mistake. The ones I sent are brightening up the nurse's station nearby…

-GERALD

E-mail—Tuesday, June 27, 2000.
Subject: Lynda Status—Day 89

They finally pulled Lynda's trachea tube and she is tolerating solid food! She is asking for her glasses and books.

They are talking about sending her to the rehabilitation wing of the hospital in a week or two, then home from there when she is strong enough. This we hear through the social worker, who couldn't say what the plan was for the leaky bile duct. I guess the implication is they expect that to heal. I guess dialysis is not such a big deal while the kidneys wake up—she is creating some urine but not enough.

There is still a ban on flowers—apparently routine with transplant patients.

The boys and I are visiting through 4th of July—anyone who wants to visit later in July should check with me about the local family housing unit, as the rate is going up!

-GERALD

E-mail—Friday, July 7th, 2000.
Subject: Lynda Status—Day 99

The boys and I visited over 4th of July weekend. Lynda was able to ride a wheelchair and beat us at cards—definitely getting stronger and clearer of mind. Yesterday they were able to place a "stent" or tube through the bad part of her bile duct, so we're on the way to resolving that issue. Lynda could be in rehab in as little as a week if all goes well, then transferred to rehab near home in as little as 2 weeks—again, if all goes best possible course.

-GERALD

E-mail—Wednesday, July 19, 2000.
Subject: Lynda Status—Day 111

Lynda continues to make progress. Her bile drain should be coming out and her kidneys are showing progress.

The bad news is they have determined that her hearing loss is pretty profound and likely to be permanent. This is due to all the antibiotics she has had to take—many of which are oto-toxic (damage hearing nerve cells). Because of background noise sensitivity, speech comprehension will be a problem. Hearing aides may be an adjunct to lip reading but will not completely correct her hearing problem. We're all learning sign language and looking for other communication aides.

They hope to get her into Rehab at the transplant center either Friday (7/21) or Monday (7/24). They expect to keep her there for one or two weeks, then transfer her to someplace closer to home. I'm looking to go down to help and to learn about immune suppression drugs. I may have to stay up to a week before bringing Lynda back to local Rehab. Right now there are no out-of-town visitors scheduled from Saturday 7/22 through 7/27.

Thanks for all the support and prayers,
-GERALD

E-mail—Tuesday, July 25, 2000.
Subject: My status next two weeks.

Lynda is fast approaching the point where (we hope) she will be transferred from the transplant center to local Rehab. I wanted to alert you to the possibilities regarding my absence from meetings scheduled 8/7-8/8.

I intend to take family leave for at least some portion of Friday 7/28 through Monday 7/31 for a visit, then return Friday 8/4 to be with her on a scheduled check-up, probable removal of the bile duct drain. I'm hopeful that I can drive Lynda back up here either that weekend or early the following week. Depending on the findings and how slow things work, I might be back to work Monday 8/7, might miss that day or three, or might have to postpone that trip to another time. It all depends on how well Lynda is doing in Rehab.

The business meetings on Monday 8/7 and Tuesday 8/8 are my concerns. I think either could be done without me, but if for some reason it is imperative that I be there, we may wish to be prepared to reschedule. Sorry my crystal ball isn't any more clear.

-GERALD

E-mail—Tuesday, August 1, 2000.
Subject: Lynda Keep Status—Day 123

Visited Lynda this weekend—she is doing remarkably well in many ways. She has thrown herself into the physical therapy (she gets 5+ hours daily) and can now get up from the bed into a walker (with the slightest of boosts and a steadying hand for balance) and make it across the room. She can get from a wheelchair into the car almost without help—in fact we ate at restaurants twice! We also wheeled our way through Wal-mart with gown & mask flying…She was able to point her big toe up yesterday for the first time.

Her hearing is virtually gone—starting slow progress on lip-reading and finger signing. Kidneys doing a little bit but not near enough yet. We hope to put the bile duct issues to rest at the end of this week.

One MD's guess puts her at 2 weeks from being able to go home, if she continues on as she did at the transplant center. On the other hand she could get more visitors (very important to her right now) if she transferred to rehab back home, but that might set her back a bit (an extra week?) A hard choice—and one she may not have to make depending on what the Docs say.

Stay tuned—and thank you for your support!

-GERALD

E-mail—Monday, August 7, 2000.
Subject: Lynda Status—Day 129

Lynda is heading back to the hills of Appalachia! She will make the long ambulance ride *Thursday* 8/10 and take up residence (for a couple of weeks?) at our local Rehabilitation Hospital. Very exciting! She is of course thrilled.

-GERALD

E-mail—Friday, August 11, 2000.
Subject: Lynda Status—Day 133

Lynda has arrived in the at the local Rehab hospital and is in good spirits, though her ears are playing tricks on her, which worries her. A bunch of doctors and nurses lined up to wave good-bye when she left the transplant center.

Lynda can receive mail (still not flowers) at the address for the Rehab hospital. Directions are easy, and the hospital is well marked. Lynda is eager for visitors (still need gloves and gown), though they try to keep the patients busy and try to restrict visiting hours to:

4-9 Monday-Friday
1-8 Saturday
8-8 Sunday
Permits to leave the facility possible on weekends.

Lynda can't use the phone and doesn't yet have e-mail, but you can call the front desk or you can reach the nurses station. You might wish to call to make sure we don't have Lynda out painting the town or something if you hope to visit on the weekend (though our older boy has a soccer practice Sunday at 4:00).

How long until she gets home is an open question—I'm betting on the week of the 21st—just as school starts for the boys. Time will tell.

-GERALD

Journal Entry—August 15th, 2000.

Day 137. My first Chinese cookie fortune since my counselor suggested recommencing my journaling activity: "You have an active mind and the keen imagination".

◆   ◆   ◆

E-mail—Tuesday, August 15th, 2000.
Subject: Lynda Status—Day 137

Lynda is doing well at the local Rehab hospital—has skipped the last two rounds of dialysis. They're watching her numbers closely, but this seems to be a turning point! Good morning kidneys!

She is off VRE isolation status but is fighting a staph infection in her wound, so visitors still need gown & gloves—I'd say a small step forward there.

The doctors are talking about sending her to the house Thursday 8/24. Lynda is talking about Tuesday 8/22 if not sooner, so we'll see who gets their way!

I will go to the hospital tomorrow morning to learn about her PT/OT exercise regimes, which she will continue to need on a professional basis at home (outpatient) for awhile.

-GERALD

Journal Entry—August 24th, 2000.

The human-resources people at work have this idea down pat—it is so important to have short-term goals and a sense of steady forward progress. This keeps you functioning day to day.

It means however that each climax is a "false peak" with a bigger mountain beyond. You then are in danger of sinking into despair at the larger task facing you—perhaps you lost that important short-range goal. It's all an expectation game.

This is how it was over and over again. What's the difference between a series of healthy short term goals and "one damn thing after another"? Anticipation, expectation.

The home stretch is a classic example of this.

We were at the rehab Hospital near home—Lynda eager to get home and the docs willing because of "all the help" she would have (I did it to myself again?). We were scheduled to leave Tuesday morning 10 to 11 o'clock a.m. but got a call Monday evening saying Lynda's blood count was low, and she needed a transfusion in the morning. Fine.

Well they couldn't get her blood to cross match that evening—four sticks and she said "enough", so next morning they're still trying to type her. I warned them about the extra factor that had slowed down our surgery.

They ultimately went to the dialysis port for the sample but had to call many times to figure out how the central line worked. It was some sort of thing with antibiotic reservoir that had to be drained.

Anyway Lynda's just steaming as the hours drag on. The plans for boys' soccer practice were in kaleidoscopic change. We agreed to have me come back after practice to get her and arranged for a neighbor to take the boys in. They didn't get started until 5:00, so plus two hours times two units plus one hour observation meant after 10:00pm.

Then I got a call—Lynda had a reaction to the first unit of blood—temperature and blood pressure spike. They want to stop the transfusion and hold her until the morning.

Fine—call the neighbor and thank her for her willingness to help—catch her next time.

Well, Lynda was outraged. She felt she promised the boys (and herself) she was going home today and refused to cooperate further—refused medicines and everything—wanted to go home. The nurses called and described the "difficult situation". I agreed to come get her but only on the condition that she cooperated with them to make this as safe as possible—take her medicines etc.

The workers were very nice—even locked themselves out of the hospital in their efforts to help us to the car. I had had to use the cell phone to get their attention in first place—offered to call inside for them—they said no problem—somebody was coming, so we left the three of them standing outside in the dark parking lot and headed home. Arrived 10:30.

Problem was Lynda had runs—bathroom had no safety rail (windowsill no good), and the seat was too low. I definitely had to help her up and down to the bathroom every 30 minutes through the night. I think I got three hours sleep that night.

After being rescued by the CNA, I took the boys to school and headed straight to the hardware for elevated toilet seats and a safety rail, and took them back and installed them. Rush to work for urgent consultation, put out production papers for most recent crisis, and headed to a meeting with boss's boss about how to boost morale around work.

Lynda was so tired and relieved to be home she didn't want to get out of bed. Forget the chore list about arranging PT, OT, audiology test, brace molding, etc. etc.. I had to leave boss's meeting early to pick up the kids.

Also she wasn't eating or drinking, continued with the runs, and was nauseous. CNA finally got a doctor that would talk with us and a referral to a medicine that let us get through the second night—I slept—Lynda says she called twice and couldn't get me. She had changed into a nightshirt herself, but no falls.

Then the CNA calls in sick and with a sick little girl at home—time to call off work and try to get boys to school myself (big thunderstorm woke us up—with my youngest in my bed) and get Lynda in to her 10:00 doctors appointment.

Well no way could we do everything including vitals and all in one and one-half hours. She got to stay home while I took the boys to school. She said I was wasting her time (to sleep).

Worse, she was very difficult. Wouldn't let go of the wall to measure her weight—kept moving during blood pressure measurements. While trying to get a glucose reading, she kept taking the test strip out of the machine to put blood on—insisted this is the way she always did it—even though she was patently wrong, and it reset the machine. Had to get stuck four times to get machine to work—my way.

Did I mentioned the pills? She has quite a collection—two big horse pills that gag her and taste too bad to chew or put in applesauce. She lost all her bed time medicines. I could count them all in the wastebasket in clear water—so…We tried again a little at a time. Used applesauce chaser. Threw out last quarter of most foul one so as to not lose her medicine.

Now it's 8:46 and I need to put a stick of dynamite under her—10:00 appointment!

◆   ◆   ◆

15

Sound—the New Frontier

	Winter	Spring	Summer	Fall
1988	(2) Engagement	(3) Wedding		
1989	(13) Reflections on Adoption			(4) Adoption
90-95	(4) Raising our Children			
1996			(5) Swelling	(1) Christmas
1997	(5) Diuretics	(5) Dehydrated	(5) Encephalop-athy	(5) Encephalop-athy
1998	(5) Encephalopa-thy	(5) Encephalopa-thy	(5) On the List	(6) Holding to Family
1999	(6) Holding to Family	(7) Big Crash, Shunt	(8) Dominos Falling	(9) Live Donor?
2000	(9) Aborted Hopes	(10) Transplant (11) Closing Up (12) Lingering	(13) Beacon (14) Long Dis-tance	(14) Rehab **(15) Hearing Loss**

Let me tell you about the devastating effect of a total hearing loss. Okay, Lynda could hear an air horn by her ear or a jet plane landing on her head. Anything less and she heard nothing—80 to 100 decibel loss across the frequencies.

It didn't help any to consider the choices—her hearing was taken by the same antibiotics that saved her life, so there was really no choice. She was suddenly isolated and alone in the "sound of silence".

Oral communication is the obvious first thing you miss. The first thing I did when I learned that Lynda would have a permanent hearing loss was go out and buy every book on sign language I could find. There is quite a range, including dictionaries, phrase books, and books on grammar and language from the perspective of a person deaf at birth. The way they "establish space" in constructing pronouns, for instance. This is American Sign Language, which I found fascinating and inspiring, but of course Lynda was coming from the same side we were—newly deaf and grounded in spoken English.

I felt the responsibility to learn, and be a life-bridge and support for her, so greatly that I would literally lie awake nights practicing. I needn't have worried; it turns out that it is much easier to learn to finger-spell than it is to read it. This was especially the case as Lynda had to deal with her loss, psychologically, before she could gear up to really seriously learn. As a result, she put off the idea of classes, and I was the one to teach her most of the early sign-word vocabulary that she got. If I didn't know a sign, it didn't matter because she didn't learn it. Any sign language she had learned before surgery (more than I had for sure) was just gone.

I also looked into portable keyboard devices, but the convenience just was never up to good old paper and pencil. I wrote a *lot* of notes.

Other basic essentials of living were quickly missed. Telephone is the most obvious one. Lynda's contacts through the Special Education network quickly introduced us to the VCO or Voice Carry-Over telephone. This device lets Lynda talk and be heard normally, but the incoming voice is translated by a communication assistant and shows up on a liquid crystal display on her VCO. This translation service is offered for both incoming and outgoing phone calls free of charge. This was truly liberating. Only problem was, she couldn't hear the phone ring (and early on couldn't walk to it even if she expected a call). Similarly she couldn't hear a doorbell or an alarm clock. There are devices you can buy that translate these signals into flashing lights and vibrating beds. We haven't invested yet, but I see those as necessary steps towards independence.

Driving is another one. Apparently you can drive deaf in our state with a special sticker on your license. This means you can't hear horns, sirens, or squealing brakes, but perhaps this doesn't matter. She's getting stronger as I write; driving will come soon enough.

People scoff at how much television has come to dominate American culture, but the point is, it has. Miss one, you miss the other. And what is television without the sound? Not much. Note that Radio has survived, but picture-only TV has a rather limited following—mostly security guards.

The answer of course is Closed Captions, those little letter boxes that try, sometimes successfully, sometimes not, to relate the dialog and sound effects that the rest of us hear. Even the best of them simplify the sentence structures, and of course inflection is lost. Virtually all the broadcast TV has CC now; I'm amazed though that companies spend $2.3 million per minute on Super bowl commercials and don't always bother adding CC's—which can be a blessing if you hate commercials as much as I do.

Most movies you'd rent today have CC's, but golden oldies from the 60's or the days of black and white are lost to the deaf, unless they've developed such a cult following that they've been re-released. Classics like "It's a Wonderful Life" are now available close-captioned. Musicals—I suppose they try, but why bother? I'm surprised how many non-fiction educational films still don't have CC's—no budget I guess.

What hurts the most along these lines is first-run movies. No public theaters put closed captions on the Big Screen. When our boys want to see something new that's all the rage—The Grinch for instance just came out that season—Lynda is left out.

Hard to compare that to the pre-surgical experience of trying to get her to screen Star Wars Episode I when it first came out. She was slightly encephalopathic and had the runs due to the lactulose she was taking to flush out the ammonia, and spent most of the movie wandering around lost in the theater. What a trade-off!

We used to enjoy a night out at a dinner theater. This is out of the question now, followed by Symphony and other concerts.

But what really hits home the hardest for me is the loss of music in the home. Lynda used to enjoy music, and drew particular comfort from the relaxation CD's that I brought her as she coped with pain and misery before surgery. But music wasn't a real big part of her life; she was discouraged from performance early in life.

My upbringing on the other hand was the opposite. One grandmother was a music teacher and played piano for the silent movies when they were new. My mother sang to us children constantly. Everyone else in the family played piano as well as other instruments—my meager mastery encompassed only saxophone, tuba, recorder, and guitar. At my peak in High School I was taking 4 out of 7 classes in music, both performance and composition.

Music was crowded out of most of my college and early work years. The exception was International Folkdance, which is incidentally how I met Lynda. Our dancing days are over now; you can't dance if you can't hear the music.

We wanted to give to our children all the best things we enjoyed as kids. This was part of the responsibility we took on as parents, and, to me this included, of course, Music. I did the singing to the children as infants. Our school system had a simple music program in elementary school. Among the last things we did before the surgery was take our oldest boy to the advance music placement night to choose instruments for the beginning of middle school in the fall; our efforts to secure a suitable trumpet were interrupted by the transplant, but were completed before Lynda came home. She went to his Christmas concert that winter because he was proud of his accomplishments; this was his very first concert, and he wanted her there. But of course she could only tell there was music because I tapped my foot. It was so sad—she was still using the walker, and of course with parking and getting in and all we were late and had to sit in the back of the auditorium. We could barely see the band, let alone our boy.

I had been trying to get our youngest interested in music, and I knew with his limited attention span, the most music for the least effort would be had from today's electronic keyboards with all the bells and whistles. Lynda had resisted the idea summer of '99, but I was on my own for his birthday summer of 2000, so I took the plunge. A keyboard is actually much less expensive than a trumpet, but it more than balanced out, in the little guy's mind, the big bucks we were spending on his brother's instrument.

Playing the keyboard together was one of the bonding things I did to get back together with my sons when I returned without their mother. Only later we got the word—she would never hear the music he could make.

There were other never-agains to deal with. One of Lynda's favorite things, and one of the few that she collected, was music boxes. I had actually gotten her no less than three Wizard of Oz music boxes for her birthday that spring. She spent her birthday in a coma that year, but later as she came around she delighted in the sparkling Emerald City water globe that played "We're Off to See the Wizard" and took solace from the Ruby Slippers globe that played "Somewhere Over the Rainbow". I would tell her those Ruby slippers would get her home yet and play the song for her as she lay in her bed with IV's, catheters, and breathing tube through her trachea. She'd be so happy. Then the next day, with her short term memory wiped clean by the drugs, she'd be happy to receive such a wonderful music box all over again, clinging again to the hope of some day getting home.

She'll never again listen to those music boxes, or the Mouse on a Dreidel at Chanukah, or the Carousel ponies, or my favorite, the one that plays "The Rose". Raindrops and Roses and other Favorite Things went the way of the dog's bite and the bee's sting. A cochlear implant may let her recognize speech again, but, as I understand it, it will lack the tonal discrimination necessary to enjoy music. Never again.

I had looked forward to the day when the boys would develop enough musical savvy to enjoy caroling at Christmas—another of my childhood memories. Instead, I'll have to look forward to gathering the family around the card table. Many games will be too hard without speech, but most of them we can manage to make fun.

And she can enjoy watching them play soccer. Our youngest just discovered wrestling, and she's insisted on coming to watch his first practices and match.

Life goes on; we will find things for our family to do. But, they won't be the same things I enjoyed most as a child—not and include Lynda. I feel like I've irrevocably lost that piece of my childhood, and won't be able to pass it on to my own children. Like the Von Trapp Family in "Sound of Music" but reversed. Curse this disease for stealing music away from my family.

16

The Saga Continues

	Winter	Spring	Summer	Fall
1988	(2) Engagement	(3) Wedding		
1989	(13) Reflections on Adoption			(4) Adoption
90-95	(4) Raising our Children			
1996			(5) Swelling	(1) Christmas
1997	(5) Diuretics	(5) Dehydrated	(5) Encephalopathy	(5) Encephalopathy
1998	(5) Encephalopathy	(5) Encephalopathy	(5) On the List	(6) Holding to Family
1999	(6) Holding to Family	(7) Big Crash, Shunt	(8) Dominos Falling	(9) Live Donor?
2000	(9) Aborted Hopes	(10) Transplant (11) Closing Up (12) Lingering	(13) Beacon (14) Long Distance	(14) Rehab (15) Hearing Loss **(16) Home Care**
2001	**(16) Bile Drains**			

Journal Entry—August 26th, 2000.

Well, after a day and a half of "the Runs" we got her on Imodium which stopped it, but the pain stayed. Friday all the CNA could get in her were her medicines, three peanut butter crackers, and 8 ounces of water. She hurt a lot, so we consulted and headed to the hospital.

Left the boys with a friend.

After taking copious medical history the doctor checked with the transplant center, and the (upsetting) idea of going back there was brought up.

Best guess: it was a flora and fauna die-off in her intestine which left it to be colonized by a less friendly bug.

Nothing was to be decided until morning so I left 9:30, ate horrid food from Hardee's for supper (onion rings that had were chewy and tough, and a dry sandwich with under ripe tomato that didn't agree with me), and got the boys. In the morning we packed up the boys for five soccer games this weekend. (Later they added a sixth). Our youngest is going with one family for two games in another city while the oldest is going with a second family for a game downtown. Then that family will get the youngest if need be, keep them both overnight, and take our oldest to two games on Sunday.

Got to hospital about 10:00 a.m. after touring the back roads to our friends' house—almost like a road rally—"2 1/2 miles across bridge then turn right at the grocery bar". Lynda was just being wheeled out for a sigmoidal endoscopy. All of the overnight tests—blood, urine, X-rays, and stool were normal, so it's not the presence of a bad bacterium. It could be a viral infection—different test. Could be absence of a bacterium, maybe, that should be more abundant? We wait here with bated breath while they checked her out.

They said five minute procedure, but it took longer to write this than that. Allowing hospital time for in and out—hmmm—must be interesting in there.

◆   ◆   ◆

Journal Entry—September 4th, 2001.

The colonoscopy showed a few red spots, which they biopsied, but nothing obviously "wrong" in a big way.

Later, we learned, the stool sample results were not back yet. Ultimately it turned out to be a C. Difficile infection. This opportunistic little bug likes to move in and take over when antibiotics have cleared out the normal flora and fauna in the gut—this is apparently quite common. My initial reaction to the runs of feeding Lynda yogurt was on the right track—if only she was able to eat much.

The treatment for C. Difficile is usually Flagyl—which Lynda is allergic to. The second choice is vancomycin. They put her on a two week course of the vancomycin, and she perked right up. All that lying around and moaning was for a well defined specific reason. If only we had put our finger on it sooner.

I chuckled to note that the treatment was really based on the stool sample results, and the sigmoidal endoscopy was for insurance only. Cover their asses by probing hers? I suppose they might have found something.

The vancomycin is actually another oto-toxic one, but they assured us that taken orally, very little would get into the bloodstream, so she shouldn't have any further deterioration of what's left of her hearing.

Lynda's allergies to Penicillin, Cleocin, and Flagyl probably had a big impact on what antibiotics could be chosen for her, especially when the vancomycin resistant enterococcus (VRE) got into her bile duct leak. You could draw a direct link between allergies and the resultant antibiotic choices that took her hearing. I seemed to remember vancomycin IV's.

Lynda responded so well to the vancomycin that we debated the need for her to be rushed down to the transplant center for a follow-up. Ultimately they said yes (figures, doesn't it?), and insisted we be at blood draw by 12 o'clock and Radiology by 12:30 so they could examine the bile duct via contrast X-ray dye study.

We agreed to go thinking that a) they might remove the stent and drain if leak was gone, b) we were supposed to be flushing that drain daily with saline, and since we haven't been—the plastic was an infection threat and needed to be replaced.

No one told us about any special preparations, but once we were on the road I got to thinking that before procedures they usually had Lynda go N P O (no products orally?). So I got on the cell phone trying to get somebody at the transplant center to ask, and eventually left a pager message for the coordinator on call "re: Lynda, NPO???"

We got no response on our side of the cell phone dead zone in the Appalachians, and had no messages waiting once we were over the mountain. So, we figured no need for NPO and Lynda had a hamburger at 11:30 a.m.

We were on time to the blood draw lab where they took seven tubes (2 sticks and a pediatric butterfly needle—Lynda has no veins left).

I heard them answer a call while we waited, saying yes they'd have "her" in there by 12:30 p.m., so the pressure was on. They were only five minutes late. Then we got to Radiology and the "hurry up and wait" began. About 1:30 p.m. they finally got around to discovering that she was not NPO.

"No sedatives for six hours after eating," says the nurse. But-But-But—

So now ensues the great debate about what they were actually going to do today, and whether they could do it later that day or had to wait for next morning.

Now all this time, Lynda who can't hear anything, is moaning that she doesn't want to stay the night. I'm wondering if we're going to spend two nights at the transplant center since the coordinator had insisted it was an overnight thing.

One nurse thought they were just going to shoot in some dye and take a picture. I insisted that they were going to have to remove the stent via going down the throat and up the stomach like I was told, that it would require sedation and half a day to do the job—as I had been told.

The resident came in and said they would be removing nothing or everything, since it was all one piece. I said that seemed unlikely since the drain and the stent were put in at times two weeks apart. He went away to check and came back to assure me it was all one piece now.

Anyway, they decided we needed to come back in the morning 9:30 and called it all off. We were to be NPO this time, no guarantees when we'd get out of there. We had a follow-up with the surgeon who basically confirmed what I thought. He said we can't flush the drain Lynda had in right now, but that we needed to be set up to flush it in the future.

Turns out the Prograf (anti rejection) medicine blood test was no good since it was not a morning "trough" value, found just before taking the next day's dose. So we needed to get another blood test the next morning 8:30 a.m. for Prograf, then take only the medicine we absolutely had to, then go on NPO status (vancomycin, Prograf, prednisone).

At this point it was quite clear I would not be home Friday in time to take the boys to the soccer tournament six hours away that Labor Day weekend. That's six hours in the opposite direction from home as the transplant center. So Auntie, who thought she was coming to stay with Lynda, got to be the one to take the boys to the tournament. Well, next morning things went off without a hitch—she was in and out of Radiology in less than an hour, no sedative needed! The original nurse was right—they just shot in the dye, saw that everything looked fine, put on some serious pressure and saw no leaks, left in the one piece drain/stent combo, and called it a day. Lynda was done before she knew it.

Apparently we *could* flush this plumbing with saline—the surgeon thought it was plugged for some reason—possibly he thought we were not flushing it because we couldn't, when in fact we were not flushing it because we were not told to.

Actually, Lynda had been told to flush it, but in her mental state, she was not in charge of her own care, and that meant nothing to her. Besides, we were never given syringes etc. for the flushing.

All those delays and no sedative—we could have done it all yesterday and left! At least Lynda got her wish and didn't have to spend the night in the hospital—she stayed in the hotel with me.

We had an "accessible" room which seemed no different from others I had stayed in except they put me on the second floor for the first time. I suppose there was a railing in the bathtub, which she couldn't use anyway given the hole in her side.

Mailers—mailers are white cardboard boxes with stuffing in them for mailing in blood tubes. We need these to send in for Prograf levels—this being a test the local labs cannot do.

Lynda was supposedly given a dozen of these which she was sure she gave to the rehab Hospital. I had them search, and they came up dry—perhaps she gave them to the rehab people at the transplant center?

The coordinator said she'd mail some—which we never got. The second set of mailers got there the morning we left for the transplant center.

They were kind enough to give us a half-dozen more at the transplant center, so now we have plenty—but have not yet used one in our home state.

Perhaps the hardest thing on me during this time is Lynda's attitude. She had enough regimented activity at the hospital and invasions of her privacy to last forever.

So, when I try to wake her in the morning, she rebels. When I gave her the list of all the things we needed to do—thinking I was being a help by organizing—we instead get in to a big argument—how dare I do this to her?

I have to point out that, yes, someone's life really might depend on doing these things, that I had watched her fight infections the last five months that nearly killed her, and which did take her hearing. It IS a big deal that she falls asleep with pills on her bedside table. A regulated four times daily medicine is less effective and gives worse side effects when you take them sporadically and virtually double up.

Figure 1. Drug Level Over Time, Depending on How the Pills are Spaced.

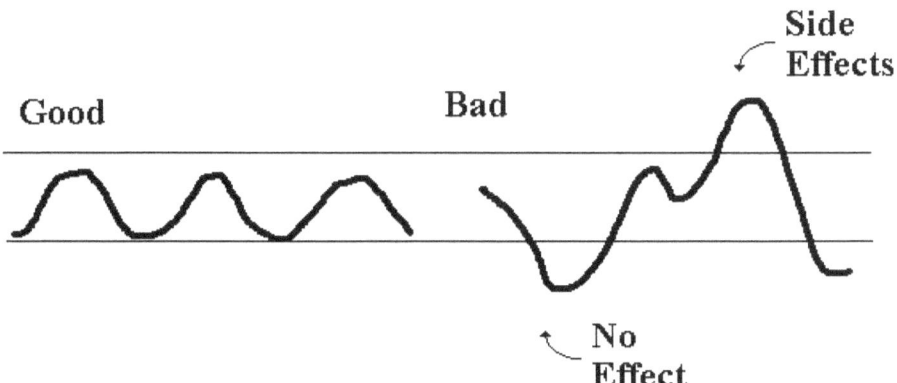

We *do* need to flush the lines and we *do* need to change the bandages.

We're getting almost everything done now, but it's very hard on me. I feel like I'm doing something for her and look for some gratitude, but instead she makes me feel like a monster for pushing pills on her when she's trying to enjoy dinner or when I intrude on her with questions about bandages, metrics (blood pressure, weight, temperature, blood sugar), or bowel movements.

She says she knows what needs to be done, but it is still only getting 90 percent done with me doing a lot of pushing—less if I don't.

And I'm supposed to be inspired by what to keep pushing? Where do I get energy to try to help someone who basically resists me for doing it?

Note: she no longer has the excuse of encephalopathy! Back then, my efforts were keeping her out of the hospital. Little voice said—OK, stop trying so hard, let her steer, and if she proves she can't by crashing, she's back in the hospital and no longer in your care, (until transplant, anyway)

Now, that logic doesn't even hold water, since we'd just be back where we are today at a given point on the road to recovery. I'd have the same job to do over again so letting her crash now could only make sense as a permanent thing. It's all or nothing right now—if I'm stuck with her, I can give no quarter and must keep pushing.

A friend who works with the deaf came over and introduced us to voice carry over (VCO) telephones and the network communications assistants. I wonder if they are paid or volunteers?

Lynda was thrilled to finally be able to converse and acted like a little kid—calling everybody to show off her new toy.

Too bad AOL connections are so crappy in this area—I finally canceled our service—we need to get e-mail back—except more reliable than AOL ever was.

◆   ◆   ◆

Journal Entry—September 5th, 2000.

Lynda is getting better day-by-day. She seems to be able to keep track of what's going on and is in many ways herself again. She's throwing herself into PT and developing serious leg muscles.

She is OK in the house by herself—she spent half an hour (asleep) 45 minutes between the CNA leaving and us picking up, and is now tackling an evening soccer practice (2 hours) with just our youngest boy in the house with her.

◆   ◆   ◆

E-mail—Friday, September 8th, 2000.
Subject: Lynda—Procedures
Dear Transplant Coordinator,

We had another interesting (and potentially dangerous) glitch we need to discuss.

When we first noted Lynda's high blood pressure on Wednesday, we called the local GI doctor for advice. He said we really needed to start taking such things to a regular doctor—it had been years since he dealt with things like blood pressure—and that we should call the family doctor who we saw at the local Rehab hospital, and has been recommended as a regular internist. However, he said that if we can't get hold of that doctor, go to the ER and somebody would see us.

Several messages were left with the family doctor with no result on Wednesday, and her blood pressure stayed high. Lynda really resisted the idea of heading into the ER, since we weren't clear on how high a blood pressure was really "critically dangerous" vs. simply a chronic problem, so we started looking through the literature from the transplant center. There we found the statements about blood pressure being "consistently" above something over 85 (on the daily measurement program) dictating that we call in. We settled on paging the coordinator on call, got your relief Wednesday evening, who passed the baton to you Thursday morning.

You did a great job getting us set up with a prescription, calling it in, letting our CNA know what to do—she went in and got Lynda on the stuff around lunch time. I went in that evening to pay for those prescriptions, and was surprised when the pharmacist said, "We have another one called in here for you."

"Oh really," I said, "what is it?" Blood pressure medicine. Same as this one we already got? No, Altace. We talked about the bio-mechanistic differences. Who called it in? Somebody with the same first name as you, about 3-4 o'clock.

Hmmm, I thought, the transplant coordinator has been really working overtime. At which point he dropped the other shoe—the Doctor's name was not from the transplant center—it was the local family doctor. Best I can figure the family doc never got the messages Wednesday night, probably got them first thing Thursday morning, probably set up the orders then, and the nurse took until mid afternoon to get it called in. I've checked with the CNA, and checked all our answering machines—we never heard back from them directly (and wouldn't even know the prescription had been called in if I hadn't dropped by the pharmacy).

This is obviously a dangerous situation, with two different doctors calling in prescriptions via two different nurses, both with the same first name. If they had been two hours quicker, Lynda might have been taking an unintended mixture of blood pressure medicines. The root cause of course is that we're not clear on what sort of issues to take to which doctor, and consequently opened up more than one door here. The family doctor doesn't seem to be positioned to deal with "emergent" issues quickly, but we hate to call the transplant center about a hangnail. We're on a bit of a hair-trigger here and don't know which way to jump.

Please give this some thought, and let us know how we should be screening and directing health-care concerns here.

Thanks,

-GERALD

Journal Entry—September 19th, 2000.

—blood pressure high—medication—Pandora's prescription
—blood pressure too narrow
—eating poorly—stomach problems again and nausea
—blood count low 19.7 vs 22 last week and 27 the best she's had. She's got two-thirds the red blood cells she should have!
—appointment to talk with the doctor tomorrow.

◆   ◆   ◆

Journal Entry—October 5th, 2000.

Well, here we are in the hospital again.

Well, the doctor ordered a stool sample and a CT scan with contrast back on September 20th, also the Iron study the nurse had suggested, and stool sample.

The CT scan contrast was a nightmare for Lynda—if she could drink four liters of chalky suspension, she wouldn't need the CT scan. Note: the liquid sort diluted with Kool-Aid is much better for a nauseous patient, even though they have to drink more.

By about Wednesday we had our first office visit with a new family doctor. No result on CT scan yet, but stool sample was negative for everything tested—except that they didn't test for C. Difficile. Had to do that one again.

By Monday we were scratching our heads over the CT scan results—colon not swollen, fluid in abdomen, and enlarged spleen. This we got informally over the phone—our GI doctor was waiting for the transplant center to take the lead, but they never got what he sent them!

Monday night 3:00 a.m. (Tuesday morning really) Lynda called out, and I came downstairs to find her sprawled in the hallway with blood everywhere. I used her nightgown to mop up the worst of it and threw it in the sink, turned on the water, then administered first-aid. A one inch crescent shaped cut on her left big toe was the source of most of the blood—the really nasty one was her left hip—a scrape or tear about 8 inches long and a big swollen hematoma. It actually wasn't bleeding much, but when I put a piece of gauze on that, it was hard inside.

She insisted she wanted no doctors involved, but that hematoma really looked bad. I got her a new nightgown (2), mopped up the water that had run over from the sink, and called up our neighbor to come stay with the boys in case they woke up.

We went to the ER where they X-rayed her hip. While we were waiting, I found a marble sized bump on the back of her head. At first she argued that it was an old bump and wanted me not to tell the doctors, but of course I did. She eventually admitted it was a new bump when she couldn't lay her head down flat any more. She showed no sign of neurological distress, so the bump on the head went untreated—although it all turned blood red over the next few days.

The X-rays showed nothing broken and no internal bleeding, so in essence they put Neosporin and Band-Aids on the two wounds, and sent us home.

All this because Lynda went to the bathroom herself, stood up from the wheelchair, tried to change her nightgown, and fell backwards, hitting her head upon the chair and twisting her leg (I guess the toes struck the metal bed frame).

The hip turned into a giant bruise with bloody oozes that wouldn't clot off for days.

Tuesday we were scheduled to go to the transplant center to have the bile drain removed but her leg was so sore she didn't think she could travel, and we postponed the trip a week, setting the stage for two to three more disasters that followed as a consequence.

Lynda's Monday blood work showed low white and red cell counts, and so more blood draws were ordered for Wednesday (would not have been if we'd gone). The results showed continued decline in the red and white count and a shocking ten-fold reduction in her platelet. Her GI doctor was so concerned that he called us himself and insisted we come into the hospital right away—with no clotting factors a simple fall wouldn't clot, and she could bleed to death. So, we called around, arranged to drop the kids with our friends and headed in.

Repeat of the blood work (lady hit blood first stick) showed platelets were normal again—the early result was probably a lab error with decimal point shifted.

The doctors were still concerned about the low CBC panel, so planed transfusion in the morning, cross matched her, and were all ready to start in the morning. I went home to my own bed.

I woke and called in, only to hear that Lynda was refusing the transfusion. I went into the hospital instead of work to find out why she had refused another transfusion. Lynda said she wasn't refusing anything, and said the doctor had said the transfusion was completely optional—though I heard different from the doctor. Best I can figure Lynda had started out insisting that she wanted go home and put the doctor on immediate defensive. We had a long and spiteful argument until Lynda ultimately agreed to have the transfusion rather than risk another flaky blood test on Saturday that could lead to her missing our older boy's birthday party. She accused me of blackmailing her and implied that I was a bully who wanted to run her life and tell her what to do, just for my own ego.

Somewhere in this whole deal the CNA's mother was hospitalized so I had to go get boys and call back to see how the transfusion was going, while trying to plan whether to bring the boys or what.

Surprise! Four or five nurses working together couldn't get the transfusion started. Ultimately the first lady came back and hit it again—transfusion didn't get started until 5:30pm. I discussed choices with the boys and they decided that rather than being dragged around in the car in the middle of the night, they would just stay home all alone in their beds.

I finished baking a birthday cake (in the form of a Star Wars Episode One Trade Federation Droid Control Battleship), put the boys to bed, and fetched Lynda back from the hospital about 1:00 a.m..

The birthday party, at a Laser place, was a great success, with 16 kids, two siblings, and three adults playing Laser Tag. We'd pulled off another one for the boys.

Well, fall weather started getting cold, and we all developed sore throats and runny noses. Monday, Lynda started running a fever that slowly crept up during the day. The CNA got her to the lab for a blood draw but couldn't mail the Prograf test kit in because it was Columbus Day. We were scheduled to have the bile duct removed at the transplant center Wednesday, October 11th anyway, so we decided to carry it.

Lynda's fever rose to 101 degrees while the CNA was here, and we debated what to do. Couldn't get hold of the GI doctor for the Monday follow-up we were supposed to do per release instructions. Ultimately called the transplant coordinator and discussed options. Could go to to ER on Monday if bad or take her in early Tuesday to the transplant center's ER to see their GI doctors. We decided to do the former if the fever got worse, the latter if it held steady—and sent the CNA home.

Not only did Lynda's fever jump to 102 degrees, but she started leaking bile from around where the drain left her side.

And so we called up our friends who gamely revised their plans, we packed up for a week, dropped the boys, and headed into the transplant center in the middle of the night. Several stops—some for toilet, some for dry heaves—and we got into the transplant center ER about 2:00 a.m.

In the E.R., an ugly scene developed in which Lynda was in total denial that she needed medical attention. She insisted that she did not want to stay in the hospital. She wanted to go sleep in the hotel, and wait for the scheduled Wednesday procedure and Thursday G I clinic—this while unable to eat or take her pills, and having repeated dry heaves.

She flat wouldn't believe me that for bile to get from the liver to the exterior of her drain it had to pass through her peritoneal cavity, and so her abdomen was probably filled with bile. This would be the mysterious "fluid" seen two weeks earlier on the CT scan. The pressure probably explained the bloated feelings and lack of appetite. If it was infected, that would explain the fever.

It finally took several doctors to convince her that she was serious enough to need to do it now—though she was still not happy with that. The whole situation was my fault, I had talked her into being here, and she didn't appreciate it. Amid the usual "you do the procedure then", and complaints about trying to sleep, and not resting in hospital, she asked me if I had ever slept in a hospital. I avoided the retorts that I had done it quite often—usually sitting up in a chair in her room. Nor did I mentioned my time not sleeping so that she could sleep, like the previous night, or the post procedural semi-sedated times with breathing tube in.

It is so hard to care for and about someone who fights you, fights the doctors, and is a general pain in the butt!

◆   ◆   ◆

Journal Entry—October 26th, 2000.

Here we are at the transplant center again, mainly to have another go at pulling the drain out of Lynda's bile duct. It has been a glitchy weird trip indeed.

Five minutes before we left yesterday, our oldest boy called saying he missed the school bus to our friends' house, and he and his friend needed us to give him a ride, so our departure was delayed half an hour or so. After we arrived at the school and put the boys in the van, our friends pulled up. They noticed the boys' absence when their girl showed up without the boys. (She didn't bother telling her Dad about the boys missing the bus—he had to ask).

We spend the night in the motel, pretty uneventful except that there was no safety rail around the toilet. Lynda tried for it anyway, and I followed her in the middle of the night just in time to catch her as she fell, trying to transfer from the wheelchair to the toilet.

We got relatively lucky with the morning blood draw, and so had 15 minutes to catch the bus over to the ambulatory care center for her 9:00 bone density scan.

Well, the lift on the bus didn't work to get the wheelchair in, so they had to call a special van. The new driver didn't even know how to work his own straps. We got to the place where the scan was to be done, about 8 minutes late, rode the elevator to X-ray, and were told we were in the wrong place. When they changed Lynda's appointment date, they had also moved her back to the main hospital!

On the return trip, the bus driver tried to call the wheelchair van for us, but it was not available. He ended up loading us on the bus (this one's lift worked).

We were back to X-ray in the main hospital half an hour late. Lynda thought we had canceled the task, and wanted to wait until 10:30 to change her gown, so there I was in the large woman's dressing room writing her notes about why she should take her clothes off, while another lady sat nearby with advice about where to find the gowns.

We finished the bone scans and were actually five to 10 minutes early to vascular Radiology. We were sitting there in the lobby/atrium waiting area, Lynda in a gown and blanket on her wheelchair, when the X-ray tech came and told us Lynda had moved too much (was hard to explain the importance of not moving, when she couldn't hear). We had to do the scan again.

Fortunately Radiology was in none too great a hurry to get started on Lynda. We've been waiting a half hour now...

...We were just told the procedure was delayed because someone came into the E.R. with a ruptured aorta and that takes priority–but we are still on for today.

...1:19. Well, they still haven't removed the drain! They replaced it again! She will be asleep awhile (half hour?) so we will be late to G.I. clinic—late getting rid of the drain—late for everything! Let's just put our whole lives on hold for a while longer!

Turns out Lynda has a ball of hardened gunk (unidentified) hung up behind a constriction in her bile duct. Now the plan is to return again tomorrow a.m. and have them put in place a double diameter drain. Then in a week or two or more they would go in and remove the ball of gunk.

So we called up the CNA who talked with our friends and negotiated how to divvy up the child care arrangements, and we headed back to the hotel—via a restaurant.

We chose Greek for my second meal of the day and Lynda's first. We got there at 4:50 and they didn't open until 5:00 according to the sign. We waited until 5:10 and still saw no sign of it opening, so we changed plans again. We went to a seafood restaurant. After standing by the ladies room door for 10 minutes while Lynda negotiated the wheelchair to a toilet, I had salmon and Lynda had fried oysters—about four of them before she had to rush to the restroom again and toss her cookies. So much for a pleasing $44 dinner. We ended up in the exact same hotel room, though we can have it only the one more night due to "Parents' Night" this weekend at both the local universities. So let's hope tomorrow holds no surprises, and we can head home after five to six hours observation after the 7:30 a.m. procedure. All they planned to do was place bigger tubes in the openings already in her biliary system—no new cutting or anything

◆   ◆   ◆

Journal Entry—Sunday, October 29th, 2000.

The procedure went well, and they did not need to observe her any longer than the two hours it took her to wake up.

We ate Greek finally, and she was all spacey and weird. Happy. Then she slept all the way home—five hours nonstop.

She slept all Friday night (except for a bathroom trip or two) and slept most of Saturday except three hours at the soccer mini tournament. She was awfully confused and irritable. This continued through Saturday night. She was very weak and unable to shift her weight—needed lots of help to stand up.

During the night she asked me to take her temperature—she was shaky—wanted cranberry juice. She was running one degree of fever.

This morning she spilled her cup of ice and juice all over the floor and peed in the bed. After getting cleaned up, her temperature was 100 degrees in her armpits.

I called the transplant center to page the coordinator, called off the barbecue we had planned with old friends from my school days that had come to our town recently for a faculty position at the University. Too bad—we haven't got together since they moved here, and I was so looking forward to it.

I need to keep pushing on the transplant center, and take Lynda's temperature again. Don't know whether it's a case of "take Tylenol and watch" or rush her off to the transplant center or local emergency room or what. Aaaargh!

This is getting real old.

◆   ◆   ◆

E-mail—Monday, October 30, 2000.
To: Transplant Coordinator
Subject: Lynda Status—The Adventure Continues

We spoke to your colleague on Sunday about Lynda's fever spike (hit armpit 100.6) and sleepiness/confusion, and she advised us to head to an ER for blood cultures. We took Lynda to the local hospital on Sunday afternoon.

Lynda's fever basically went away, but she has trouble staying awake, and is somewhat confused and disoriented when she is awake. It is almost as if she never completely threw off the anesthesia from Friday's bile duct dilation. She can't stay awake long enough for you to write a response to things she has asked, misses words for a few things, has somewhat sluggish speech.

So far she is negative on ammonia and acidosis—blood cultures are yet to return anything. She has tossed her cookies twice that I'm aware of—Saturday afternoon and Sunday evening. She has no unusual pains or complaints—wants to go home and doesn't think she's sick (but then she wouldn't).

Her blood counts are back down around the 20+/7+ level again. Platelets 44K. Just barely into the dehydrated range. Blood pressure is fine.

The family doctor has seen Lynda. The local GI doctor (or his on-call) will be visiting Lynda late this afternoon to get his read on it. The nurse didn't anticipate Lynda checking out tonight, and of course we all really want to see the results of the blood cultures.

I wasn't sure if the local Docs were keeping you informed of events—wanted to let you know in case there is anything else we need to do. Doesn't look like we'll be taking her into the lab for the usual blood tests/Prograf check this week.

Thanks,

-GERALD

Journal Entry—Monday, October 30th, 2000.

Well, yesterday afternoon we took her into the emergency room on the advice of the transplant center coordinator.

All the initial blood work turned up negative—ammonia, acidosis, etc. only mildly dehydrated.

Her blood count was down again.

Her temperature recovered to normal.

However, her speech remained slurred; she was disoriented and very slow on the uptake. Not just me but also a friend that visited and the nurse as well.

The doctors breezed through and basically said, "she has no fever, she's not throwing up, she can go home as far as they were concerned!"

I had to discuss Lynda's symptoms with the doctor, particularly her inability to stay awake. He agreed to keep her overnight and look in to it—saying that he hadn't noticed.

I realize that this is so draining because it is a throwback to the days of encephalopathy. I have particular bad memories of those times when Lynda's mental function was a crapshoot and it didn't look like we'd be able to control it at all. This is like that—Lynda's not altogether there and the docs don't even recognize the problem, let alone know what to do about it. When the Doctors don't even have a plan, one feels very, very alone.

Review

8/22	checked out of the rehab Hospital a.m.a.
8/26-28	hospital with intestinal problems, C. difficile #1
8/31-9/1	transfer to transplant center during soccer tournament
9/9-11	weekend? Monday? Hospital?
9/19	blood pressure in play
9/20	GI doctor visits
9/27	CT scan
9/28	family doctor visits
10/2-3	fall—emergency room visit to local hospital—mobility problem cancels transplant center visit
10/4	night time—low platelet count, transfusion
10/5-6	in hospital with C.Difficile, #2 treatment
10/10-12	transplant center—bile duct leak
10/16	visit to the nephrologist
10/25-27	transplant center—bile duct dilation
10/29, 30, 31	local hospital admission for confusion and fever

Next: transplant center—cleaning of bile ducts

◆   ◆   ◆

Journal Entry—November 1st, 2000.

Just talked to the family doctor. Lynda has C. Difficile for the third time and also bacteria growing in her bile duct.

He is still consulting with an infectious disease guy, but what they're trying to do is establish what the threshold is for sending her back to the transplant center.

The odds of releasing her free and clear before the weekend are nil. There is a low chance of transferring her to the transplant center before the weekend. Nothing generally happens on the weekend itself, so the most likely case is that we'll be looking at her on Monday, November 6th, trying to decide if she should go home (i.e., is responding to antibiotics) or should go to the transplant center then.

If they decided to let the antibiotics run a cycle, that would take another two weeks, which is when they wanted to do her bile duct cleansing procedure anyway. So we are either looking at home, or the week of November 6th for another run to the transplant center, or waiting until she gets over the infection before she can do the procedure. If this runs into Thanksgiving, I might have to follow her to the transplant center the week after that because of course everybody has plans.

The family doctor is also concerned about her nutrition—this might correct itself if they can cure the C. Difficile, but it needs attention.

◆   ◆   ◆

E-mail—Wednesday, November 1, 2000.
Subject: Lynda Status—Day 215

Lynda is now angling for the 8th hospital admission since returning from her 5-month hospital stay post-transplant. Most of the trouble has revolved around C. Difficile in her gut (a bug that likes to move in when the normal flora and fauna is killed off by antibiotics), and efforts to restore her bile duct to proper function—she still has a drain in her side. All this has prevented her from eating well and has slowed her progress in terms of strength—her blood count is low, and she is still mostly using the wheel chair. Her hearing is a total loss, but her kidneys and liver are doing their job.

I can't even keep track of all her visits any more, so for anyone who needs a handy reference list, here goes:

8/22	Checked herself out of the local Rehab (0) after a reaction to a transfusion—day 144 of her initial hospitalization.
8/26-28	Local hospital (1) with first C. Dif caused intestinal problems.
8/31-9/1	Transplant center (2) worked on her bile duct drain
9/11	I missed work on family leave but can't recall why now (2 & 1/2???)

9/19	Lynda went on medication for high blood pressure
9/27	Outpatient CT scan due to continued intestinal trouble
10/3	ER visit to local hospital (3) 3:00 am after Lynda falls in wheelchair transfer—lots of blood and big bruises but no stitches
10/4	Night—we're called in due to what probably amounted to a bogus lab result—dangerously low platelet count
10/5-6	Lynda stays at local hospital (4) for transfusion and begins 2nd round treatment for C. Dif
10/10-12	transplant center (5) for more work on bile duct
10/25-27	transplant center (6) again for more work on bile duct—this time dilating a narrow section that was holding up a hardened blob of gunk
10/29-11/1	Admitted to local hospital (7) with fever spike, confusion, and sleepiness. Has C. Dif for a third time and infection in her bile

Next—whether she goes to the transplant center (8) directly in the next few days or sometime in the next week or two (perhaps after visting home briefly next week) to remove the blob of gunk, that's the next stop!

Keep us on those prayer lists—the "adventure" continues.

-GERALD

Journal Entry—Monday, November 6th, 2000.

It's been difficult to get the whole story from doctors. At times they seem to be neglecting major aspects, but things seem well on track.

They weren't concerned about borderline dehydration because of all the fluid swelling in her feet. As that went down, they finally started her on IV fluid Sunday.

Bile is naturally dirty stuff; there is no compelling reason to react to finding bacteria in her bile drain.

Lynda's mental function has waxed and waned in terms of sleepiness, vocabulary, complete sentences, disorientation, and having vivid dreams that are mistaken for fact later on. Because of the erratic nature of the problem, and Lynda's tendency to put on a good face for the doctors, it was very hard to assess. The nurse finally put it to me bluntly that malnourishment and dehydration were the cause. Sunday, Lynda was much more clear but rather depressed about her prospects—the nurse recommended an aggressive schedule of PT/OT etc. to focus her mind and get her stronger.

The neurologist consult turned up "over compensation for hearing loss" as a factor too—she reads more into lip-reading then she should and goes off on these tangents due to what she thinks she heard.

Lynda understands the effects of malnutrition from her work with kids and understands her discharge is predicated on her eating well. She calls it blackmail—with a bit of a smile.

◆   ◆   ◆

Journal Entry—November 14th, 2000.

I'm kind of sad that we didn't even decorate for Halloween. I feel like that's a big thing that slipped. We put up a skeleton on the door (with black light), and that was it. Lynda was still in the hospital, so we did do trick or treating in the traditional way—on a more populated road with our friends. Nobody seems to have come to our house while we were gone (not much candy missing) so we have three buckets of candy. My will power isn't what it used to be.

Lynda has been home all week now, doing pretty well. They put her on vancomycin for 30 days this time to really nail the C. Difficile.

Lynda's prime problem now is depression, despite the medicine, so she doesn't have much appetite, or energy, or initiative to do much. She acts as if all the sign language we worked on before is all new to her, and doesn't show much interest in learning. She both wants company and wants to be left alone—no serious discussions. She fights against eating and against taking her pills on our schedule. Very draining

Also more than one fecal accident—hard on us but hard on her too—very much. On a rational level she sees her life as a mess and doesn't take much joy in anything, or see the point in working things out.

◆   ◆   ◆

Letter—November 20th, 2000.
Dear Lynda,

I am writing this after your 5:20 a.m. bout of vomiting. I'm very sorry you don't feel well. You said the medicine went up before it got down, so I take it this means you don't know whether or not you got this dose of Prograf down—7 hours after I gave it to you.

The plan with Prograf is to take it on a regular 12 hour schedule, which relates to the half-life of the medicine. It jumps up when you take a dose then slowly fades to a lower level just before the next dose. If the low level is too low, your liver will start to reject, just like if you skipped it completely. If the high level is too high, you suffer side effects like high blood pressure (possible bleeds) and lowered immune system response (more colds etc.). We hope there is a window where, with discipline, you suffer neither of these bad results. If your medicine comes at a poorly controlled schedule, you may end up with both sets of problems.

It would be dangerous to get your Prograf level checked at the lab this morning, because the Doctors would prescribe a change in medication based on bad data. If you really did hold down your Prograf, then you wouldn't really be at a 12-hour low. They might improperly lower your dosage too far, setting off rejection. If you did NOT hold down the medicine, then you would be on a 24-hour low, and they would improperly raise your dosage and increase your side effects like blood pressure.

You ask me why I'm always getting mad and pushing pills at you. This is why. Playing games with Prograf is self-destructive. Somebody had to die before you could get their liver and somebody else may have died because they didn't get the liver you did get. I think you understand the responsibility this lays on you.

You want more sense of control? This is it—you can either take control over your pills or not. I have failed to keep you on schedule and can't keep pushing you in these circumstances.

See if you can get back on a good pill schedule today, so that you can get a good check at the lab tomorrow.

Still here, still loving you,
    -GERALD

Journal Entry—December 10th, 2000.

The transplant center visit went fairly well. Before the procedure I helped to get Lynda where she needed to be, into a gown, etc..

They gave her sleepy drugs, and then tried to get her to roll over to another table on her belly. Since her eyes were closed and she couldn't hear, that was a real struggle. Then they had to put a bit in her mouth so she wouldn't bite the endoscope. She of course fought that in her dream state, and nearly bit the nurse. I had to help hold her during this.

Later when we were home she asked me if I still "wanted her". I pulled something from my counseling sessions and told her that I was playing too many roles. I had just had to hold her down while they put a bit in her mouth, and now she wants me to make love to her? Slow down! I can't change hats that fast. This perspective helped her a lot—she said of course she doesn't like that it's that way, but this has helped her understand.

They removed her external drain finally, but still had to leave a stent to hold open her bile duct. We'll go back January 4, 2001 to either change it out (it will plug up) or remove it completely.

Yesterday, she told me she found two lumps between her right breast and her armpit. Of course she is now very upset over the notion of having to deal with cancer. She has had a benign cyst in that area before—it may even be the same cyst and her just being so skinny that she can feel them easier. She was down to 109 lbs. She used to look boney when she was below 130 lbs. a year ago.

I don't have the emotional energy to react to this last development. One more thing, one more chore is how I feel.

Lynda says it can't be cancer because one person just can't have that much bad luck.

Not and live through it, I think to myself.

◆   ◆   ◆

Journal Entry, December 29

Last days of the first 2000 years AD and we're finally seeing someone about Lynda's toes.

Upon discharge, she was still so swollen we had to buy her jumbo size shoes. As her protein intake went up and her albumin stabilized, the swelling went down but her big toe nails had cut sideways into the fleshy part of the big toes, where they were squeezed by the other toes. We didn't pay a lot of attention since we were focused on her bile duct and central wound care.

However, infection set in, and as she began walking (without even a cane now!), she was limited by the pain in her big toes.

I realized they were in crisis only when I was hit by a rotting smell, and discovered the first joint was all purple on both toes. This was about 2 weeks ago now—we've been soaking in Epsom salts and pouring peroxide on them at least once daily since then.

Today we're seeing a specialist to try and get it under control. They're better now, but at the worst point they made me think of gangrene and possible loss of the toes!

Despite that, her walking is getting better, and my heart doesn't always leap to my throat as she totters along like a penguin. The thought of a fall and busted hip putting her in the hospital another 6 months is not pretty to contemplate.

◆   ◆   ◆

Journal Entry—January 4, 2001.

At the Transplant Center this morning to have the stent in her bile duct removed or replaced, hopefully the former. Lynda is in good spirits, despite pain from her toe nails, and is walking around, mostly with just a cane or nothing.

They removed a lot of "stones", "gravel", and "debris" after dilating her bile duct with a balloon. They put in a different type of drain—will return in 3 months to clean out more and remove the tube. The endoscopy specialist is pleased with the results. "Two or three more sessions and she'll be done," he says. Second session would be 1 month after the first so April, and May.

◆   ◆   ◆

Journal Entry—February 1, 2001.

Lynda is doing very well. We went back to the toe specialist a second time—Lynda had a big toe nail removed each time but we have the infection under control now. Lynda is walking without a cane, and wearing shoes (her oversized ones because of the big bandages on her toes). She's eating—no more C. Dif infection—and she's getting stronger.

Better yet her spirits are improving. She's cooking and trying to help around the house, and is actually pleasant to interact with for a change. It's not all misery—she's more at peace.

The hearing loss is all that's slowing her down physically (curing PTSD will take longer). No pain, no overwhelming fatigue. Life is looking up.

◆   ◆   ◆

Journal Entry—February 26, 2001.

Lynda continues to do well. She's climbing stairs, talking about driving, and getting stronger.

We've been visiting her counselor together, but I didn't need that to know how much emotional investment I had wrapped up in getting a new computer system. It included

- Lynda's promise when we got her diamond, the symbol of becoming dependent with the computer equalizing accounts and symbolizing a return to partnership.

- The one thing Lynda did to "promote my personal growth" per our wedding vows was support my writing. My bad feelings about the lost creative side of my life was tied up with her returning to support my writing.

- General feelings of sacrificing my life for the short term and setting up the computer as the reward at the end of the rainbow.

I kept trying to justify the purchase of a really good one, talking about her use in e-mail, our oldest boys' need for internet at school, and so forth.

She resisted over spending so much money and quibbled. This just made me more and more indignant until eventually I told her that I thought she just enjoyed the power position she was assuming.

She said no, she just wanted me to admit that I *wanted* it, which I did, and we were in business.

Yesterday I set up the internet connection and showed Lynda what it could do. The first thing she did was go to her university web site, look up the page on the programs she had built, and checked out the staff listings.

She was not listed. Her face fell and she slumped. She said, "I want to get out of here," and quickly retreated back to her bedroom.

I tried to cheer her up, but there was a tear in her eyes as I tried different approaches—that they were protecting her privacy, or that she needed to get strong and go set them all straight (as she was refusing breakfast).

What she finally said was, "It's time for me to go back."

◆   ◆   ◆

Journal Entry—April 18-19, 2001.

Returned for a flush of her bile duct. Stent replaced (actually a twin was replaced by a set of 3 with dilation).

The SNAFU for this time—we were scheduled for an ultrasound right after endoscopy. Well, they couldn't do it, because the bowels fill with air during endoscopy, and this blocks the ultrasound imaging. Next time we do the ultrasound first.

Return in 3-4 months.

◆   ◆   ◆

17

The Effect on Me

	Winter	Spring	Summer	Fall
1988	(2) Engagement	(3) Wedding		
1989	(13) Reflections on Adoption			(4) Adoption
90-95	(4) Raising our Children			
1996			(5) Swelling	(1) Christmas
1997	(5) Diuretics	(5) Dehydrated	(5) Encephalop-athy	(5) Encephalop-athy
1998	(5) Encephalopa-thy	(5) Encephalopa-thy	(5) On the List	(6) Holding to Family
1999	(6) Holding to Family	(7) Big Crash, Shunt	(8) Dominos Falling	(9) Live Donor?
2000	(9) Aborted Hopes	(10) Transplant (11) Closing Up (12) Lingering	(13) Beacon (14) Long Dis-tance	(14) Rehab (15) Hearing Loss (16) Home Care
2001	(16) Bile Drains	**(17) Reflections, Me**		

Some nurses have their eye clearly on their jobs, and obviously are making an effort to control their irritation at visitors who might be in their way. Policies about formal visiting hours encourage this view. The better nurses recognize that the visitors can be a big help in caring for patients—indeed their presence can have a great impact on the patient's recovery, and these folks will be the primary health-care providers after the patient is discharged. Thus, involving and educating the visitors takes on a certain level of importance.

The best nurses recognize that the patient's health is under a microscope, and that the patient will get the best care possible. But also, the patient's family is experiencing a stressful crisis without anyone looking after them, indeed that the patient's primary care giver at home may be the next one hospitalized, possibly even as a result of this stress. These nurses ask whether you are getting enough sleep, whether you're eating properly, and in general how you're doing. They offer you soda and crackers just as they would the patient themselves.

And friends and family seem to understand this, on at least an instinctual level. Everyone seems to offer "if there is anything that they can do", though none of us can really think of anything much. They all say they don't know how I do it, and marvel that I am holding up so well under the stress.

As a matter of fact though, my health is being slowly sacrificed to achieve the goals I have my eyes fixed on; I am slowly bleeding it away as the cost of bringing my boys' mother home, and keeping life as close to normal as possible for them. Sleep, avoidance of fatty fast food, time to relax my blood pressure, creative outlets, even dedication to career, all are put second priority.

But at the center of it all, beneath the level of the deliberate sacrifice, is an awful gnawing horror that resulted from seeing my love and my life's work destroyed before my eyes, and being helpless to do anything about it. The aching emptiness I feel, the suppressed adrenaline, the frustrated desire to do something, all add up to that instinctual need for warmth and comfort and shelter we received as children when our parents made sure we were dressed, and loved, and above all, fed. On a level below our control, we equate food with our mothers love, and so the gut level response to the empty gnawing feeling is to eat. Oh, there are others—sexual overdrive, short temper, emotional sensitivity, restless lack of focus—but the one that does the damage is the eating. You eat to fill the void, only it doesn't, and you overeat. Nervous snacking, swallowing your frustration, all are names for the same thing.

My weight can be used to chart my progress through maturity under fire. At my first blush of maturity I weighed 180 pounds, and kept it under 200 all through college and into graduate school. I was neither fat nor in great shape, but I was happy and stable—big guy that I was. My first experience with being burglarized broke all that and changed my sense of security and property forever—and launched me through the 200 barrier to stabilize at 220 pounds. Leaving school to work in the real world pushed me to 230, which I held up until we got married. I was happier then, and my weight fell all the way to 213. Then came the children, and all the worries of parenthood, from the frustrations of balancing being role models and policeman, to the worries of protecting them.

When I hit 250 I started having "undercarriage" problems—knees twisting on steps, heel spurs, sore feet as never before. Shoes off the rack were never comfortable again. It took three years to recover from probable cartilage damage to my knee without surgery—plus a dedicated effort to control my diet, that stabilized me at 240.

Then Lynda's trouble started. Each new hospitalization would be accompanied by another jump up in stress, and another jump up in weight, and at my worst I broke 280. It affects my digestion, and I have run through eyeglass prescriptions at a record rate. I started in on low doses of blood pressure and cholesterol medicines to keep things in the normal range, and then later doubled that, and doubled the blood pressure medicine again. As of right now I'm down to 275 lbs., but my blood pressure is still reading 150 over 105 when I get home from work.

It's not like I don't understand how I'm supposed to eat—and actually think I do very well qualitatively.

There are several different schools of diet philosophy; I learned to appreciate several different ones. In the end, though, there was no denying the latest government studies and its basic grasp of the obvious—if you overeat and under exercise, you're in trouble.

If my physical health is deteriorating, my mental health is worse. While in one sense nothing happened to *me*, in another sense a lot happened to me. My wife was taken away, my children were traumatized, my house was let slide unchecked towards decay, my career effectiveness was interrupted, and all extracurricular activities were put on hold. No part of my life was untouched by these events. Now, how can I looking at anything I might do or build and feel a sense of satisfaction, because everything has been shown to be vulnerable to the capriciousness of our health? Everything I've worked for has been muddied in some way—how can I complacently forget events and go back to what I was doing before?

What I have is classic post-traumatic stress disorder (PTSD). I'm in a constant state of alert attention, trusting nothing, relaxing for nothing. No wonder my blood pressure is in play. First thing in the morning, before taking any blood pressure medication, my resting blood pressure—best it can ever get during the day without drugs—is 145 over 105. All night my arteries are above the magic number 90 so are losing their elasticity, setting me up for a coronary. Maybe this whole thing is killing me, literally.

So what's the emotional defense to all this? Either a) find a solution, or b) stop caring. My efforts to find a solution are never ceasing—perhaps so and so can join us and provide our family with security—but that doesn't just happen. Nothing is so easy.

So must I turn my back emotionally on my wife in order to survive? What about my worries for my children, who have been damaged on deep psychological levels by all this? Must I distance myself emotionally from them in order to survive? If I stay for them, will the stress kill me and traumatized them even worse? None of these answers is acceptable—I can't just abandon everything I've worked my whole life to achieve.

Sex is only a minor factor in this. Our sex life has suffered for at least five years and has been virtually nonexistent for two. Now Lynda looks like a cross between my grandmother and a concentration camp survivor, though she's getting stronger all the time. But I can't even kiss her without wondering whether I'm passing her the germ that will ultimately kill her—how can I resume a sex life with this woman? Forget the nightmare visions of her laid out semiconscious with a dozen tubes in her—how can I ever make love to her again? This is just one more little casualty along the way. Also she is emotionally blocked at showing any empathy for my problems, because the mere act of recognizing them sets off guilty feelings in her. The deafness inhibits communications, and pillow talk seems impossible. I guess my only hope is to somehow convince myself that celibacy is not the booby prize for long and faithful service. Society does not recognize sexual outlets for people in my situation.

My day job took some strange twists too. I mentioned the simple distraction of not being there, or having to schedule around the family, curtail business travel and even social functions. A more insidious effect is that the mundane routine seems so trivial and unimportant now. It's hard to get motivated. My most productive moments seem to be when ambition wanes so much that doing mundane tasks in a mindless way seems a relaxing balm for the stress. Usually my trauma drives me to seek clear meaning in the big picture type activities, strategic planning. I'm good at that sort of thing, so my vision quickly outpaces the organization's ability to follow my lead—or perhaps it's a lack of authority in my position. Frustrating either way. I'm ready for career change, but who's going to promote someone to a position of increased responsibility when they're cutting back to 40 hour weeks, or less with family leave, and are never sure if they will be able to keep an appointment? Some times I want bigger and more glorious responsibility, and other times I want to climb in a hole and hide. I have never been known for my tact, and I have had a bit of a bulldog tendency, forcing people to address the root of a problem. But as my patience disappears, diplomacy goes with it, and I find myself alienating people I shouldn't. This is a problem—the company has been very good to me, and forgiving on the whole, but there are limits.

There are some good sides to the experience. While my knowledge of the depths of hell has grown, so has my confidence and skill in coping with everyday challenges that others might find daunting—as indeed I once did. Changing wound dressings, IV lines, flushing out bile duct drains, giving shots, inventorying pills, and providing disabled access are all taken in stride. The daily circus of scheduling medical visits, dealing with which kid needs to be where, who is sick (mine or the CNA's), who'll be driving Lynda where, and so on, has become quite complex—but routine. I miss few birthdays of nieces and nephews, but never have been any good at thank-you notes. I've taken responsibility for directing CNA-type employees, and have no doubts about my ability to care for the kids' basic needs all alone (psychological needs are another matter). Indeed the routine is easier with Lynda not home, quite the opposite of what all my acquaintances expect.

The big one though is that this has forced me to consider again what is important in life. The little things, the day-by-day, are they castles made of sand or the only thing that matters? Is it the quality of life or the footprints that we leave behind to echo through eternity that matter? Raising children no longer seems such a slow sure avenue to improve the world. With confidence in everything undermined, the big bold bids for immortality seem more attractive. I feel the loss acutely of the lost creative arts in my life, and I look forward to the day I can retire and write. If such is successful, and touches enough lives, there is a security in numbers that is not threatened by the capriciousness of our health.

We're mortals, and can be snatched away at any time. What will we leave behind? What kind of people will we have been while we were here? Does caring for the sick or disadvantaged, like Lynda, consume our lives or make us better people for having done that? Many people have told me that they have found courage in our example. That is hard consolation though when you feel so alone, so isolated, in a place beyond the understanding of the people you see every day. And that's the hardest thing—the isolation, the loneliness. It's not so much a matter of needing to be held—this has proven that I can cope—but of needing comfort. The world is a scary place, as it turns out, and we're not getting out of here alive. We need someone to hug us and care for us, and show understanding—and someone we can do the same for. That person once was Lynda—perhaps again, but deep down I don't think I can believe that any more. Maybe I'm too scared and hurt to let myself believe again. Perhaps the final casualty is our hope and faith.

18

The Effect on the Kids

	Winter	Spring	Summer	Fall
1988	(2) Engagement	(3) Wedding		
1989	(13) Reflections on Adoption			(4) Adoption
90-95	(4) Raising our Children			
1996			(5) Swelling	(1) Christmas
1997	(5) Diuretics	(5) Dehydrated	(5) Encephalopathy	(5) Encephalopathy
1998	(5) Encephalopathy	(5) Encephalopathy	(5) On the List	(6) Holding to Family
1999	(6) Holding to Family	(7) Big Crash, Shunt	(8) Dominos Falling	(9) Live Donor?
2000	(9) Aborted Hopes	(10) Transplant (11) Closing Up (12) Lingering	(13) Beacon (14) Long Distance	(14) Rehab (15) Hearing Loss (16) Home Care
2001	(16) Bile Drains	(17) Reflections—Me **(18) & on the Kids**		

We all felt bad about what this situation was doing to the boys. It was not like a single event though; rather the effects of a sick parent built slowly, and progressively popped up in more and more aspects of their lives.

With both parents having careers, our boys were probably in a better position to weather the storm than if we had had a more traditional division of the work to begin with; such as one with a career and one taking primary care of the children. Since we took equal roles in the childcare, we were able to keep the basic services going long after the point where a "traditional" family would have fallen apart.

The boys were already used to their mother disappearing on a business trip for a few days or even a week. They knew the rules and expectations each of us set, and they were in many ways easier to care for with just one parent around, because they weren't tempted to play one of us off against the other.

The first phase of the illness that impacted this equilibrium was when Mom was too "tired" to play with them. Whether it was indeed fatigue, or sore feet, or nausea, or back spasms, or depression, or drug side effects, Mommy simply needed a lot more rest than she used to. In a child's world, this meant that Mommy wasn't much fun any more. Then of course when she felt better, she would over-compensate with wild enthusiasm, spoiling them rotten and under-mining my efforts to maintain order and discipline over homework, chores, bed-times, manners, etc.

Even when Lynda was undeniably sick, and really couldn't get out of bed, this wasn't anything too remarkable in a kid's life. Children in school bring home every flu bug that passes through the community, so Lynda and I regularly were laid out by the same bugs that the boys themselves experienced. These were times for overt sympathy, flowers, breakfast in bed, or the loan of a favorite stuffed ani-mal until Mommy "felt better".

The first few times Lynda showed obvious signs of Encephalopathy were scary, but the boys soon learned to deal with it. They would come to me and say, "Dad! Mom is being weird again!" Sure enough, they sometimes alerted me to signs of an onset of some sort before I had noticed. Over time, our older boy even got so he could laugh at her a little, then would take a surprisingly mature objec-tive role as observer in tracking her behavior.

When Lynda was in the hospital for short times, it was really not that big a thing to them—Mommy away or sick was routine, and "out of sight" was "out of mind". They'd occasionally miss her and wish she was here for some event or other, perhaps feel slighted that she was not there for a birthday.

It was not until Daddy had to go be with Mommy that their lives began to fall apart. They had to go sleep with friends—exciting at first but it got old quickly. Sometime grandparents came to stay with them and *they* were no fun at *all*—even more strict than their own parents! The boys would whine and beg me to come home, in ways that they never did when just one parent was missing. This made them stop and think what it might mean to lose a parent, and the worry began. They began to ask whether Mom would be okay, and the oldest let his imagination get the best of him. The youngest became clingy and huggy for the first time in his life—maybe this experience actually did him some good, opening up a softer side that had been buried under his childhood attachment problems and veneer of Attention Deficit Hyperactive Disorder.

Both boys would get preoccupied and lethargic—the Zombie boys wouldn't get excited by mundane things like preparing for a soccer match, or getting to school on time. Such things simply didn't have the highest importance in their lives any more.

The difference between the boys became most striking at the point where I had to tell them that their mother was really sick, so bad that there was a chance she might not make it.

For the oldest, it hit him like a hammer blow, but was quickly assimilated. He could discuss the situation rationally, and move on to questions of how it would happen and what would happen. Clearly the agony of continued, prolonged uncertainty had been taking a heavier emotional toll on him (as it was on me) than would be felt by facing the actual loss.

The younger boy dealt with the worst news the same way as he had dealt with the merely bad—he protected himself with denial and avoidance. After being told she was dying, he'd ask the next day if she was getting better and any minor rally turned into a rejoicing that it was all a mistake, and everything was back to normal.

I was faced with a really hard question at the beginning of the year 2002, when it seemed very likely that Lynda would be facing a very dangerous and desperate experimental surgery. There would be a strong chance that Lynda wouldn't make it through, and I had to decide how to handle the situation with the boys.

We three guys were all at home, with Lynda 4-5 hours away at the Transplant Center. There were a few days before the decision was to be made—enough time for a "final visit" before the surgery. Lynda was lucid, reading books, even had the where-with-all to give the nurse a message for *me* in anticipation of my daily phone call. On the other hand, she had a feeding tube up her nose and an IV tube in her jugular that was oozing blood because of the anti-coagulants, as well as an assortment of catheters, monitors, and simpler IV's. This is not the final image of your Mother that you want burned in your brain. The automatic reaction is, "Of course you should take the boys for one last visit," but is it really in their best interest, or is it best to leave them with better memories?

Then there is the question of whether to tell them that their mother was facing life-threatening surgery. Usually it would seem cruel to worry them unnecessarily. It would be hard to have that last visit without explaining the situation, and if Lynda passed on, the boys might ask, "Why didn't you tell us?"

Finally, there is the question of whether to let the boys actually come to the Transplant Center with me during the actual surgery. Would they want those memories of the final days of the fight to make it more real, and get closure?

The boys are different from one another, and in the end I came to two different answers. My 10-year old (at the time) had always dealt with the situation by protecting himself with distance. He wanted the barest facts, and then he wanted to be somewhere else doing something fun. He'd spend the first few minutes of a hospital visit interacting, seeing what she could do, then would glue himself to the TV. In discussing an impending return from the hospital, he only wanted to know if she'd be able to play with him. He complained most bitterly about us insisting that he get her help on homework—saying that it was too much trouble to communicate. He had always been Daddy's boy anyway.

He would be bored on the trip over, act out and be difficult in a waiting room. He would resent the restraints on his behavior—his mind carefully far away from the scary events of the day. After the fact, he probably wouldn't recognize the significance of the event or even remember the day with any special meaning.

The little one seemed best left to choose the most pleasant memories of his Mother, and be left to go on about his business of enjoying life as it came to him. We decided not only to not bring him along, but to not give him any choice in the matter so that later in life, when he takes on some maturity, he would not come to feel guilty with regrets over having "chosen" not to be there when his mother died (assuming the worst).

Two years older, my other boy was involved and hungry for information. He bonded with Lynda as an infant and was oriented towards people, engaging the attention of every adult in the room with a smile. He was seven when Lynda got seriously ill, and he not only remembers her when she was well, he followed the progress of her troubles with great concern. He was often afraid to ask too many questions, but instead let his imagination run wild with worry. You couldn't tell him just a little bit about Lynda's situation. Once he knew something unusual was going on, he'd want all the details; otherwise he would create them out of his imagination.

He was actually quite mature for a 12-year old, having had leadership opportunities in Scouts, school, and soccer. People began to tell me that not only would it be good for him to be there, he would probably be good support to me. We could do our crying together.

Ultimately, he even understood that Lynda was suffering, and that in some situations death could be a release from that suffering. He explained this to others who reported the conversation back to me.

He obviously understood the situation, and was dealing with the emotions in a constructive way. I did not worry about him like I did his younger brother, who was burying everything and would likely have to deal with the repercussions the rest of his life.

No easy answers, no single answer. Each child is unique, each situation unique, as we try to make the best out of a bad situation. I could not help but think over and over that we're grown-ups and will cope with whatever comes, but that the boys, and the damage their young psyches were sustaining, were the real tragedy in this situation.

Each of us has roots at different points on the spectrum of society levels.

I, for instance, never drew much strength as a child from the "community" level. I attended a small private school before age 10, which was followed by a move to a new part of the country and public schools where I never fit in—just at that socially formative age. Further moves associated with college, graduate school, and employment left me starting over at age 26 with no positive reference in my life to local community involvement.

Lynda's unhappy childhood was stabilized by membership in the broader Jewish cultural traditions but not by her contentious nuclear family. In fact she took refuge from her family in close personal friendships—one at a time. Her surrogate sister growing up, "Auntie" in college, and others, set the pattern, always a single individual was the focus of her social needs. This was behind her prenuptial promise to shelter me from her family. This is why when we have family or guests at our house, she tends to interpret behaviors as "picking sides" or ignoring her during the visit; behaviors she actually exhibits herself and got from her family relations.

My family experience is that of a large, very close family, that was socially isolated from the world. This large nuclear family demanded emotional closeness with several people at once and put a premium on balancing, conflict avoidance, and everyone getting along. Thus my strength and support has always been drawn from a few very close friends, as opposed to membership in a group. The number ranged from a half dozen to none at different points. Let me tell you, "none" sucks! The only society memberships that I drew strength from are abstract—and formalized: band, corporate organization, study of world religions, view of mankind's position in the ecosystem, science fiction ethos, etc.

Neither of us had the more normal experience of relating to a large body of cousins and extended family, and neither of us had roots in the community strong enough to hold us in one place.

How do people go about making friends in life? Let me refer to the "circle of closeness" concept. Each of us are surrounded by layers or bands through which a relationship will progress. The outermost layer is characterized by superficial interaction with each layer progressively more personal, and characterized by more meaningful interactions. Ideally, the process of meeting people, getting to know them little by little, progressing through the circles from small talk to deep involvement, is a gradual process with level of intimacy matched at each step to the degree of knowledge built up slowly in the relationship.

In actual fact, we tend to build walls only at certain points that represent the way that we classify people subconsciously. On a subconscious level we base this classification on the cognitive map we have of family, and society. Only those relationships we had modeled for us growing up are included in our "maps".

In my case, there is an abrupt discontinuity between family and strangers, then again between citizens and barbarians. I have a certain degree of contempt for the consuming masses but do have face-to-face politeness for a total stranger (I wave out car windows). I see those that are part of civilized society, taking responsibility and deserving courtesy, and contrast those with those that opt out (e.g. men that abandon their families), and deserve to be stamped out post-haste. For me, most people fit within the "distant polite" mode, which extends all the way in through working relationships to the wall that divides the rest of the world from Family. I function well in a corporation, with formal interactions and rules, but do not make friends easily and few people see the inner me. But, once inside my inner wall, people are welcomed with open arms and without reservation—and there is a lot of room inside that wall. It takes something like an act of malice to get tossed back out.

Lynda's outer-most perimeter is set at a cultural-values level. You belong in her world if you believe in liberal education, human rights, etc. The male "old boy network" types and scheming politicians are not welcome. She is very close and effective with groups of people with whom she shares a common cause. She builds teams. She would be a *good* politician. Most people that she interacts with routinely fit in this region, and are accepted as good friends. Deeper inside there is another wall, where you cross from the public to the private sector. Inside that wall there is room for only one other adult at a time. Displease her and there is no question in your mind that you have been ejected from the inner sanctum. However, that spot is so important that it must not be left open long, and just as quickly, peace will be made and her best friend (now me!) is pulled right back in.

This is something that has stretched Lynda's and my relationship; in my "family" view, you just don't treat others that way. All I can do is ascribe the problem to her dysfunctional family and move on.

Looking at the relationship between myself and Lynda, Lynda has squeezed me down to a "monogamous" emotional relationship with a very small circle of non-threatening friends that are not too emotionally close. This was acceptable to me when all of us were healthy and Lynda was there for me, but with Lynda's disability, and eventual loss as an emotionally supportive partner, my emotional support has been undermined, and I have nothing left. My family is thousands of miles away. My efforts to broaden this support base are taken as a threat by Lynda. Sex is a different issue—it is the emotionally close relationship with others that is threatening to Lynda, just when it is most needed by me.

Let's move on to our attitudes about childcare. Lynda does not look to the family level for the security of her children. She never had that herself. Instead she looks to the society level. With a PhD in Education, she believes in institutions such as schools, daycare, scouts, YMCA, even our network of friends. She was more comfortable than I with the idea of hiring someone to watch the kids. Now, she is in agony over the disruption her illness has caused the boys lives but still does not seem to consider herself irreplaceable, acting as if her passing on would allow us to get back to some sort of stability. She considers her disability an indirect impact on the boys rather than a direct threat to the love and support she provides them.

I, on the other hand, am acutely aware of the effect that loss of family has on the boys' sense of security and support. In their case it is further compounded by the impact of adoption issues on their development of a sense of self's position in society. At about age 10-12 they start trying to figure out their place in society, and thinking about family ties, when they suddenly realize that being adopted means some family somewhere gave them up. So then the question arises, why wouldn't *this* family give them up as well? I've felt that building a strong nuclear family support for them was particularly important.

While I did not have support at the society level growing up, I was very much aware of the lack, the fact that others had something that I did not. I envied others' ability to make easy friends. I saw my father's grief growing up in regard to the disruption our moves caused the family and our social development—he struggled mightily to get us together with cousins, uncles, and grandparents as often as possible. I watched him slide into bankruptcy with a heavy mortgage rather than uproot my youngest sister during her high school years.

I obviously look to the nuclear family to support the children, and it took a conscious act of decision on my part to defer to Lynda's daycare arrangements and reliance on institutions. I have worked hard, as they grew, to link them in to society on as many levels as possible—scouts, sports, access to friends.

Now, my anxiety and sense of failure at being unable to guarantee the support I thought they needed at the family level has been a rather self-defeating attitude as it has dragged my own health into the danger zone. I'm not much good to them if I lay myself up in the hospital or worse! But it comes from this instinctual sense of supreme importance of nuclear-family level interactions.

It's kind of ironic that given the way the boys were raised, with such diversity of interactions, they probably place less importance on nuclear family than I do!

Lynda of course doesn't see the problem. She is confident that the boys will be well cared for by *someone*, and is only worried about the problems she is causing us day by day, with her disabilities and episodes away from home, drain on family resources, etc.

So what's next? Where do we go from here?

Personally, I've got to stop trying to solve everyone else's problems and start taking care of myself. My blood pressure should be my top priority. Fortunately, with the understanding I've gained by thinking this through, I can have faith that I'm not alone, there are many sorts of help available for the boys, and *everything will be O.K.!*

I can better understand, accept, and be grateful for friends that offer to help, and can "be there for the boys" but that have no intention of becoming part of our nuclear family.

I can count the different levels on which the boys are getting support and be comforted. Between the various influences they have in their lives, they have an almost complete collection!

I can understand Lynda's needs better, and give her what she needs without compromising my own needs for friends.

My challenge: How to rebuild a network of supportive friends without disgracing myself (e.g. by letting sex slip into the picture inappropriately—all too easy to happen when you are seeking a close emotional relationship!)

Lynda's challenge: How to let me do this without feeling disenfranchised, and be at ease with the fact that building on our one-to-one personal relationship is *not* what I need in life right now. Also, how to find something meaningful to do with the rest of her life, despite her disability. She would have to do this without her customary level of energy and constant professional dedication; she would simply not be up to the effort.

For the kids, we just keep them busy, safe, and warm. We make sure they can have their friends over and participate in the activities they always have done, and are comfortable with. If Lynda passes away it will hurt them, but they have a lot of strong support, and will weather it.

19

Insurance

	Winter	Spring	Summer	Fall
1988	(2) Engagement	(3) Wedding		
1989	(13) Reflections on Adoption			(4) Adoption
90-95	(4) Raising our Children			
1996			(5) Swelling	(1) Christmas
1997	(5) Diuretics	(5) Dehydrated	(5) Encephalop-athy	(5) Encephalop-athy
1998	(5) Encephalopa-thy	(5) Encephalopa-thy	(5) On the List	(6) Holding to Family
1999	(6) Holding to Family	(7) Big Crash, Shunt	(8) Dominos Falling	(9) Live Donor?
2000	(9) Aborted Hopes	(10) Transplant (11) Closing Up (12) Lingering	(13) Beacon (14) Long Dis-tance	(14) Rehab (15) Hearing Loss (16) Home Care
2001	(16) Bile Drains	(17) Reflections—Me (18) & on the Kids **(19) Insurance**		

I can't imagine what it would be like to face catastrophic illness like liver disease without insurance. Lynda must have gone through nearly two million dollars worth of medical services. Very few people could cope with such expenses—and even for the rich uninsured, such would present a bit of a cash flow problem!

Needless to say, Lynda and I were not rich. We both received good professional incomes appropriate to our PhD educations, but on the other hand, we both left graduate school in debt, and began earning money relatively late in life. Throw in two children, and we could count our good fortunes but had little extra. We expected to pay for our children's college, but we certainly didn't have enough to cover a catastrophe. That's what insurance is for.

We were actually over-insured. Lynda was covered by a family policy through my work. She was also covered by an individual policy she had from before she was married. Since I was husband number two, and she was smart, and cautious, she had never let her personal policy go.

Both policies had a deductible which we paid, then paid a percentage up to some maximum out-of-pocket. Between the two of them, they quickly reached the point of paying 100% combined. In essence, we paid a lump sum determined by our deductibles, plus premiums on two policies. I still haven't figured out whether Lynda's premiums actually paid for themselves since either policy had a maximum out-of-pocket—the all-important safeguard vs. catastrophic illness that stood between us and a million-dollar liability.

The catch was, the insurance only paid if the claims got filed properly. Since I was also participating in an elective pre-tax commitment of part of my salary towards medical expenses, it fell to me to track all the various filings from the four of us.

In the early years, it was simple enough to keep track of the filings. I didn't even realize we could be filing under *both* insurances, so each bill matched with one EOB (Explanation of Benefits) statement that was then copied and stapled to a HCRA (Health Care Reimbursement Account) form. We never maxed out the out-of-pocket, and everything was summarized on the HCRA forms for easy reference. If I had a bill with no EOB statement, I was responsible for filing it.

The next step up in complexity came when my insurance asked if any of us were covered by other policies, and sure enough, I got acquainted with the concept of primary and secondary insurance, with all Lynda's claims going to one department of Blue Cross, then to a second department.

As Lynda's doctors' visits progressed to hospitalizations and advanced medical conditions, the providers had to do the filing, using proper medical codes etc. to justify the procedures. I could no longer take matters into my own hands by filing the bill directly.

I believe it was the provider's responsibility for filing the primary, waiting for a response, then filing the secondary, but only because they were willing to perform this service for their customers. On the other hand, it might have been Blue Cross that forwarded claims from the primary to the secondary department; in any case, it did not work well at first.

Many items got missed, so I'd get a bill and have to inquire after the filing status of a particular line item. It took two phone calls (minimum), since the two departments within Blue Cross couldn't access each other's files. I'd have to call the secondary to hear they had never gotten a claim, then call the primary and ask them to forward the information to the other department. Sometimes I had to send hard copy of the primary EOB statement to the secondary, but I got to know who to ask, and for what, to minimize the pain.

This system worked pretty well for a while with the worst problem being that my company's HCRA computer crashed, losing a bunch of filings, and they didn't bother telling us—figured we'd miss the reimbursement on our paychecks and inquire. Problem with that is that if we don't use up everything we set aside, the IRS rules say we lose it. Good thing I saved copies of everything!

After years of this Sherlock Holmes work, Blue Cross suddenly decided that they couldn't provide me with confidential information regarding my spouse, and clammed up. Fortunately we had worked out living wills and powers of attorney, so that I was able to send Blue Cross what they needed to force them to reopen communications. Lynda was in a drug-induced coma at that time.

One surprise came when a test lab decided to drop off the Blue Cross list of preferred providers, and start charging whatever they wanted. Thus we discovered the concept of "usual and customary charges", beyond which the insurance would not pay. These providers, which were contracted as Blue Cross preferred providers, agreed thereby to charge only the "usual and customary" fees worked out between them. How often when you go to a new doctor do you think to ask about their contracts with Blue Cross? Or whether their fee for a particular recommended test was "usual and customary"? I can see a consumer's responsibility to ask these questions, but in this case, we were not even the ones choosing the outside test lab to which Lynda's specimens were being sent. The lab chose to not renew their contract and the doctors, through sheer inertia, kept using them for several months. During that period, they could charge whatever they wanted without even our knowledge, and we were liable for it.

This issue was on the top of my mind as Lynda went through the process of selecting a transplant center. The one she liked best, due to the number of surgeries that they performed, their expertise, and the friendliness of the staff, happened to be out of our home state—though no farther away than the nearest center inside our state. We were in the process of petitioning for an out-of-network provider exception, when we were denied. Happily it turned out the reason was that they became recognized in-network providers via some inter-state Blue Cross agreement, in which the provider files in their own state, then the local Blue Cross sent the filings over to our home-state Blue Cross.

You can imagine how well this shuttle procedure worked, what with our dual policies, and with hers still in her maiden name. It seems that every year they changed the ID numbers too, either changing from a random policy ID number to using our social security number, or changing the alpha prefix they stuck in front of the social security number.

One problem I helped Blue Cross with was when Blue Cross paid the *wrong* hospital, and I had to lead them by the hand through a retraction and re-filing.

Our first regular pharmacy got bought out by a big chain which forced a new computer system on them. The workers were not trained, and it was like pulling teeth to get in their system. Many claims were thus lost, and I had to re-file them—and find a more competent pharmacy.

Up until summer of '99, I was able to track the individual charges, but then the six weeks hospitalization hit with up to a dozen line items in a single day. My simple system broke down. Nothing made sense until I realized that certain items were being bunched together one way on the bill and a different way on Blue Cross's EOB statement. I finally found someone at the transplant center that could print me out a detailed, day by day itemized report of the entire period, including what Blue Cross had paid against which dates, and when. It ran to eight pages. However, with a little creative matching of numbers I turned up the three dozen items that were somehow not showing up at Blue Cross, leaving me with a balance of over $6000 which Blue Cross should have paid, but the hospital was holding me liable for. These were almost all daily charges directly from the GI physicians, so were probably filed as a batch. I told the accountants at the transplant center exactly which charges our local Blue Cross had never received, and they re-filed. Again and again time passed, a bill would arrive, I would verify that our local Blue Cross had never received the claims; the center would re-file—but always through their own state's Blue Cross office. Their state office wouldn't talk with me; it was not a simple "power of attorney" issue—they wouldn't talk to mere citizens about interoffice filings.

My local Blue cross couldn't help, saying that the transplant center's state Blue Cross office should pay the center directly, and the interstate transfer was just a reimbursement procedure between Blue Cross offices. They thought I shouldn't be liable, but the bills kept coming.

A careful reading of typical hospital admission forms says we're liable for any charges the insurance wouldn't pay. It seemed I was in a trap; I could not file the forms myself (not being a physician), the insurance bottleneck wouldn't talk to me, so I couldn't force the filing to take place. I was at their mercy; their bureaucracy screws up, so I had to pay?

Some helpful clerk told me that hospitals customarily did not hold their patients liable for their own mistakes in filing insurance, but this somehow didn't make me feel much better. Those $6000 of charges were still pending a year later when Lynda went in for the real transplant, and I was able to visit with the accountants personally (no help there, though).

These claims were about 15 to 18 months old when a better glimmer of hope arrived. Lynda was out of the transplant center and going back into various hospitals every week or two with secondary conditions. Blue Cross made a big deal about "authorizing" each admission, and I received copies of all these different rulings, appeals, and reversals. I really thought that we were playing Russian Roulette with these emerging admissions until someone explained to me that if a Blue Cross contracted health care institution provided care to a Blue Cross patient that was subsequently "not authorized", they agreed *not* to hold us, the patient, liable as part of the contract. So, by that reading, if I presented my cards, and they're Blue Cross contracted, there was *no way* that I could be held liable.

Here it is now 20 months since those $6000 of lost claims were generated, and they are finally coming back as Explanation of Benefits statements (EOB's). Half say they were filed after the allowed period, and half say they are from "out of network" providers. Neither excuse for not paying is correct, but at this point I've stopped caring. I think I've got grounds for saying we can't possibly owe anything, so we're not liable, and make it stick. It's between the transplant center and three different departments of Blue Cross. They haven't seen fit to show me their contracts anyway, so I'm on the outside looking in.

Things seem to be going smoother now that Lynda has actually had her transplant. The volume of claims has of course gone up tremendously, and Blue Cross recognizes the difficulty; they assign a case worker. Thank the Lord for the resulting smoothness; I don't know how I could have sorted through all the claims. When I got home after the first two months, there were over 80 envelopes each with about a half-dozen pages of EOB statements in them.

I dreaded the prospect of sorting through these 1000 or more pages of documents, and trying to untangle the fouled-up web of cross-filings and errors that would inevitably result. I stalled and considered paying someone to help, as the pile continued to grow—the pile at least doubling in size as I waited.

I finally set out to organize them, opening all the envelopes and sorting them by date of service. Naively, I thought it would take one standard file box; it took two.

By time I had pulled out the few EOB statements that related to the boys and me, and the pharmacy claims (which were handled differently), and sorted the rest by date, I was physically exhausted. Sitting there on the floor surrounded by papers for hours, doing nothing more with them than checking the date, I had reached my limit—and I hadn't read the *content* of a single one! If five and a half weeks had generated three dozen errors worth $6000 that I might end up liable for, what would come from five *months* of hospitalizations? I was so overwhelmed by the task that I just sat there and cried; I had never felt so alone or abandoned to my fates. Lynda couldn't possibly help at that stage, and now that she was out of crisis, most of our friends had gone home. It would probably be even harder to explain it all to an accountant than to do it myself. Oh, to weather the storm only to be beaten down by the red tape!

Over the months that followed, the EOB statements kept flowing in. At one point I asked the transplant center for an itemized detail to be printed out—this was back before Lynda got home—but that quickly became obsolete (all 19 pages of it) as more EOB statements trickled in with random, spotty dates. I stopped sorting by date and pulled out only the pharmacy related EOB statements (which had reimbursement checks attached, and were needed to cover the credit card bills—medicine is expensive!) By year-end I had over two feet thick of files from year 2000 alone, half sorted, in a very full, very heavy box.

The outside service providers seemed to be getting paid, so I'm just going to let it all ride until or unless someone challenges me—and I hope my "100% coverage" defense works.

I'm making a fresh start with the New Year since I'm having to pay deductibles and file HCRA again.

I can sit down with a foot-thick pile of Patents and expect to understand (with some hard work) the twisted web of intellectual property it represents, but I was defeated by a 2-foot stack of insurance print-outs, riddled with hopeless errors and terrors, but no hope of positive pay-off at the end. It was like that video game where endless garbage falls on your head, and you slowly get farther and farther behind until it drowns you. I guess each of us finds our limits; I had never been stopped by mere busy-work before.

But life goes on, which is much better than the alternatives. The pharmacy handling changed again this year, with Linda's policy now reimbursing the pharmacist after we fork over just a co-pay. I file just the co-pay with my insurance. I didn't find this out until the first time they reimbursed my pharmacist according to an EOB statement, which I immediately assumed was a mistake. We got it all sorted out with everyone agreeing that there was no automatic transfer between the co-pay system and my Blue Cross going to happen; I was certainly going to have to do that step of the filing. But of course Murphy still rules—I've received secondary EOB statements on a few of the claims, where everybody said I shouldn't. What to believe now? As with everything else, the only answer is—wait and see. (Later: Half-way through the year, the automatic second filing stopped! What happened? No telling.)

20

Systemic Infection

	Winter	Spring	Summer	Fall
1988	(2) Engagement	(3) Wedding		
1989	(13) Reflections on Adoption			(4) Adoption
90-95	(4) Raising our Children			
1996			(5) Swelling	(1) Christmas
1997	(5) Diuretics	(5) Dehydrated	(5) Encephalop-athy	(5) Encephalop-athy
1998	(5) Encephalopa-thy	(5) Encephalopa-thy	(5) On the List	(6) Holding to Family
1999	(6) Holding to Family	(7) Big Crash, Shunt	(8) Dominos Falling	(9) Live Donor?
2000	(9) Aborted Hopes	(10) Transplant (11) Closing Up (12) Lingering	(13) Beacon (14) Long Dis-tance	(14) Rehab (15) Hearing Loss (16) Home Care
2001	(16) Bile Drains	(17) Reflec-tions—Me (18) & on the Kids (19) Insurance	**(20) Abscess**	

Journal Entry—Sunday, June 3, 2001

Things had been going pretty well for almost half a year, or up to a week ago. Lynda was driving, climbing stairs, arranging a return to work. Except for the hearing loss, she was almost herself again.

We had a lot of back-and-forth with the counselor about finding our respective muses—but that's another story.

Last week, Lynda got the flu and started with fevers and vomiting. It seemed to "break" by Friday, following a bunch of tests at the GI doctors office—(though no results yet).

Our oldest boy had a soccer tournament at a town several hours off into the mountains, and I was worried about leaving Lynda alone with just our younger boy. She insisted she'd be okay. The CNA was not going to be available over the weekend and I couldn't get any of our friends or neighbors on the phone at the last minute so I left with her assurance she'd be fine. The CNA left a pager number which didn't seem to work.

I called Lynda Friday night to let her know we got in okay, and she was fine.

I found out later that our younger boy called my cell phone at 11:16 on Saturday, but this town in the mountains was outside the range of my cell phone reception. He reported she felt really warm to touch.

I phoned about 1:30 Saturday to report the results of the first soccer games, and she seemed rather sleepy and tired. I understood that they had invited over a friend to play later in the day. Seems like an added strain but gosh, it wasn't my call.

When we got home Sunday, it was 5:30 in the evening—later than I had expected.

The first sign of trouble on getting home was our boy's semi-trashing of the house—bike in yard, Dog's electric collar off, lying in the middle of the driveway, new puppy on a short leash, which was hung up on the gate, dog poop all over in garage, inside the house there was food on the floor, evidence of playing with candles, and so on. The boys had been unsupervised, running wild.

Lynda was asleep and woke with the salutation, "Good Morning!" She was confused, lost track of time of day, didn't know that our son's friend was still there after an overnight stay. She had skipped her pills Saturday night and Sunday morning (never refilled her pill box for the new week). Surely missed Cipro, which had been added that Friday, and was not doled out in the pill box yet. I gave her her evening pills but forgot the Cipro myself.

I got on the phone and made a number of calls—to get our visitor's father to come get him took a dozen tries. I couldn't get the family where the boys usually stay. Instead I got another friend, with grown children no longer home, to come take the kids overnight. I packed up and headed for the local hospital.

Lynda was dehydrated from all the fever and throwing up. She was mentally confused, losing all her sign language, and mixing up words and generally unable to function. Probably acidosis—blood work will tell.

My worry is that her kidneys are weak and can't take more insults. The lab results showing kidney function were slightly elevated the week before, causing the coordinator at the transplant center to recommend upping fluid intake to 3 liters daily.

Is the apparent thirst and dehydration a result of some underlying kidney problem? Or could this "normal" flu-induced dry spell do further damage to here kidneys?

I got her to drink maybe 300 cc's in 3 hours. She got another 2-300 from her IV and was suddenly more lucid—woke up after returning from X-ray to announce "I'm back!" She meant, to the room, of course, but I didn't miss the symbolism.

◆   ◆   ◆

E-mail—Thursday, June 7th, 2001.
Subject: Lynda Status—Day 433

Lynda is not doing so well this last week.

Things *were* going very well, with her growing stronger and more confident every day. Then she had to fight off the flu—fevers and vomiting. This battle left her dehydrated, and we went into the hospital Sunday night. The dehydration opened the door to other complications, including pneumonia, some fluid around her heart, and possible *staph* culture from her blood (the latter might just be lab contamination, but would explain a lot if real). Her blood count is dropping, and she needs a transfusion.

Her kidneys are not keeping up with the fluid she's taking in—she has gained 20 pounds in the last 36 hours. This is not good; her kidney function was only about 30% following all her troubles last year. It's not clear she's producing any urine at all.

They are moving her to Intensive Care, presumably so they can start some dialysis.

Keep us in your prayers…

-GERALD

Journal Entry—June 9, 2001

Well, Lynda is one sick lady. She has pneumonia, STAPH in her blood stream, a falling blood count, and is making hardly any urine. Fluid is building up around her heart and pressing on her lungs. Yesterday they had to call and get my permission to change the central IV line into a dialysis port, which allows them to pull off fluid, taking pressure off her lungs so she could breath. It also makes it possible to take the poison out of her blood stream so she might have a clearer mind, and also to make "room" for a blood transfusion.

Thursday when the boys were visiting, she was quite clear and herself. I knew we had a narrow window for them to see her. Friday, she couldn't respond well enough to give permission for the dialysis. Today, Saturday, she is back to being clear but she falls asleep as she talks to you—as she did earlier in the week.

Lynda only had 30% kidney function at the end of last year—enough to function normally but no extra to spare. Kidney's don't repair themselves like a liver can. The big question is whether this episode will cause additional permanent damage to the kidneys, or will they rebound to 30% again. The IV vancomycin is supposed to take care of the staph and pneumonia.

The transplant center has called offering their support to the local hospital staff and is asking if we wanted to take her down there. I didn't see the point, but asked and learned about the outside chance of infections from bile duct blockage or leak. I promised to talk with the doctors here to be sure they were getting all the information they could from the transplant center. The local GI doctor was indeed initiating communications but was already looking out for infections and felt she was doing *fine*.

◆   ◆   ◆

Journal Entry, June 11.

The first word I got today was from the Nephrologist. He said that Lynda's kidneys were actually doing a good job of balancing salt in her blood, but that they "thought" she was dehydrated due to low albumin level. Albumin is created by the liver and its role is to produce osmotic pressure that holds the fluid in her blood vessels. He is trying IV albumin, but that doesn't have a high success rate. I'm asking whether this is nutritionally related since in other respects her liver is supposedly doing fine.

Then I get e-mail from the transplant center coordinator saying I need to talk with the local G.I. doctor—he and one of the surgeons from the transplant center think she needs to go there.

Stay tuned….

◆   ◆   ◆

E-mail—Monday, June 11th, 2001.
Subject: Lynda Status—Day 437

Lynda is back out of intensive care, now in a step-down unit. She is much more stable, and her mind is clear. The big question is whether her kidneys will kick back in, or conversely how much dialysis she's going to need.

-GERALD

Journal Entry, June 12.

The local GI doctor seems pretty certain that the albumin level is a consequence of nutrition—in her weakened metabolic state it doesn't take much to knock her for a loop. Perhaps if she starts eating again with gusto, she'll build back her albumin level.

But, due to central back pain, they've put her on a morphine pump, which she can hit every 15 minutes. If that doesn't space her out to the point of not eating any better, I don't know what will. The CNA says she ate two bites of her chicken sandwich at lunch and then fell asleep. She has this life-long fixation about her weight. She has not opened the nuts or chocolate I brought her early on. Maybe her counselor with her "eating disorder" expertise can add something here.

In the mean time, nobody has any reason they can give for sending her to the transplant center. Liver is otherwise fine, so we watch and wait.

◆   ◆   ◆

E-mail—Tuesday, June 12th, 2001.
To: Liver Transplant Coordinator
Subject: Lynda Status at the Local Hospital

Lynda is still in the hospital, probably will be awhile, probably will *not* be coming to the transplant center unless there are changes (keep us on the bed list?). I've had communications with the local GI doctor and the nephrologist—let me piece together their remarks into one picture.

As best I can tell, the most worrisome concern seems to be the swelling of the tissue around the heart which is causing rubbing. The heart muscle itself is good. This swelling could be viral or due to the infection and needs watching. It is hoped this will clear with the infections.

Her albumin (serum protein) level is low but is most likely the result of not eating much of anything for two weeks now—her metabolism isn't what it used to be. The liver itself shows no bad signs. IV albumin is being given, it is hoped nutrition will improve this longer term.

She is peeing some, not enough, but this seems related to the albumin, not further damage to her kidneys (though of course they aren't good).

She is suffering from back pain, and they have given her a morphine pump. This was a surprise to me, and seems to go against trying to get her up and eating better. I have yet to digest this bit.

Her mental function seems good, though she falls asleep on visitors and me, perhaps she's just spacey from the morphine.

Did I miss anything? If I can help you get any more information about what is going on here, let me know

-GERALD

Journal Entry, June 13.

Got a weird call at 1:00 a.m. this morning. The nurse said Lynda had had an episode of rapid and weak heat-beat, but that she was stable now. She was very lethargic and unresponsive (so was I, after being woken up in the middle of the night). The doctor had been notified and would be there shortly—did I want to be kept informed?

I said yes, as long as there was something identifiable to report—not just "we don't know anything yet". Then I couldn't go back to sleep so played computer games until 3:30.

After fully awakening in the morning, I called in to get the low-down. Turns out that she had OD'ed on morphine. With her metabolism she was not clearing it as quickly as they expected, so the 2 mg/hour dose that is normally a very minimal dose was accumulating on her. They've taken away the morphine pump, and the nurse was not clear on what plans they had for further pain management.

Later—visited Lynda at lunchtime. She was very slow and lethargic. It took her *minutes* to read a four-line note and even then I'm not sure she "got it". The things she said were very measured and thoughtful though.

She had "figured it all out"—that she was going to stay home and work on making the family a calm place. She's sure she can work out a schedule that will remove the stress and let everyone have a balanced life—allowing me to stop having to truck the boys everywhere etc. She doesn't want to have to *pay* people to play with the boys.

She thought it more important that everyone have a balanced life rather than one person getting everything they wanted.

After these pronouncements, she would sink into a peaceful sleep. I noticed disturbing things on the EKG—some patterns of two beats then skip that went on for a dozen or more, and some patterns of short spikes—double speed—about

8 in a row. Then she steadies out again. The visit was cut short as they wheeled her off to take "pictures" of her heart. The nurse said that she'd been having these odd heart rhythms—that what she had last night was different and quite worrisome. What she had today was "almost nothing"—not dangerous.

Our counselor had joined us for this visit, and we walked out together. She asked if I thought Lynda was going to pull through this time and I said I had my doubts—she did too.

What I saw was a lack of that old iron edge of determination to get out of there. She seemed resigned (though she said she had fought so hard to get out by our younger boy's birthday—two days hence). She didn't have that zest for life—she still had not opened the nuts or chocolate I brought her that first day. I opened them and stuck 'em in her face—she ate *one* peanut. She'll never pull out if she doesn't even have the will to eat, let alone the will to fight.

But, she is at peace, in a way.

◆   ◆   ◆

E-mail—Wednesday, June 13th, 2001.
To: Liver Transplant Coordinator
Subject: Lynda Update here at Local Hospital

Lynda had some irregular heat beats last night (of the "dangerous" class), which they eventually traced to overdose of morphine—her metabolism was not clearing morphine as fast as they expected when they set up her self-administer pump. This was discontinued.

Today she has had more irregular heart beats (of the "not-so-dangerous" class, the nurse says, "different") and are doing some heart imaging.

She is very slow and lethargic, without appetite, but is speaking clearly, some what euphorically, on a somewhat abstract level. She seems at peace, but it worries me that she isn't showing that iron edge of determination she used to have. Time will tell, I guess.

-GERALD

Journal Entry, June 14, 2001.

Today's update—the nurse says "not good". She has a swollen abdomen and no sound in her gut, meaning no movement in her bowels. She has had 3 episodes of atrial fibrillation, and one time they gave her medication for it. She is confused and not making full sentences, speech slurred etc. Her blood count is down again. They are going for dialysis today and will give her a transfusion as part of it.

Hopefully this will make her more clear for our boy's birthday tomorrow. But she really can't keep on like this—she needs to fight!

◆   ◆   ◆

Journal Entry, June 15, 2001.

They decided to dialyze her again today then put her on a three times a week schedule starting Monday.

However, they "tapped her out" and her blood pressure crashed. They're giving her back fluids, but she's not very lucid. Won't read lips or papers, is glassy-eyed and moaning—agitated and slurred responses to visual. She apparently stated that the doctors think she is pregnant.

Anyway, the boys don't need to see her like this, and we'll call off (or postpone) the party. Maybe tomorrow morning.

We got tickets to see the opening night performance of "Tomb Raider". That should be special for the birthday boy.

The doc writes that she gained *another* 5 pounds of fluid—we're talking 25-30 pounds total here? Or more? No wonder her abdomen is swollen, and she won't eat!

◆   ◆   ◆

Journal Entry, June 17, Father's Day.

I got a call, woke me up just after 8:00 a.m., from the hospital. Lynda's condition was worse, they were moving her to ICU, and the cardiologists needed to talk with me. She was septic.

I got hold of our friends, who could take the boys for the day, and called around.

Our oldest boy of course leapt to the same conclusion as the rest of us, said he wanted to send something to her. I told him she wouldn't know that it was there. He said he'd like to send a hug and a kiss then; I said I thought that would be a good idea.

I made sure I had my phone directory and my living will and headed to the local hospital. The father of the family I was leaving my boys with offered to come with me, but I told him he was holding up the important end of things by being with the boys.

On arrival, the Family Advocate had to call around to find what to do—then sent me in. The cardiologist was supposedly on his way soon. Lynda was moving a bit and moaning but not responsive—no sedation of any kind. Her pulse was 100-120 and not completely regular. She was sweating like crazy—temperature 100.9. Nurse said "probably" septic, cultures not back, could be the same staph.

I'm wondering how it could be the *same* one if she was getting vanco—probably pulled a switcheroo on us.

Blood O2 good—breathing in gasps, no obvious cough or rattle.

…They said she was on the maximum possible level of Dopamine to keep her blood pressure up—and it was still only 89/46.

…11:30 am. Another doctor came instead of the cardiologist. He said the fever could jump up and down as staph is released into her from an infection site or as her hypothalamus gets ahead of or behind the infection. The infection tends to suppress the operation of this system, which tries to fight off the infection by elevating her temperature. The fever breaking means *neither* that she's given up fighting *nor* that she's getting better.

The rapid pulse is likely due to the dopamine, which is given to raise her blood pressure. It is possible the low blood pressure could be due to swelling pressure on her heart or due to sepsis. It will take them up to 72 hours to culture her blood and see if there is a new micro-organism. She's not had vancomycin since 4 days ago—but they are monitoring the level and not having to replace it since she's not peeing.

The vanco might not be effective if it's a new bug but it might also be that there is an infection site that vanco is not getting into to kill the MRSA (a resistant strain of staph). I wonder whether her abdominal fluid is infected and whether the blood pressure crash sucked some back into her blood stream following the dialysis.

How can they combat such a "reserve site" of infection? How could they get antibiotic to penetrate such a cyst and clean it out?

A different doctor is now on call for the nephrologists. I will try to talk with him regarding CVC—a slow, gentle, and continuous form of dialysis.

◆   ◆   ◆

Journal Entry, June 18.

Either I'm coming down with something, have a psychosomatic link to Lynda, or this whole think is just totally mentally exhausting. I'm bone-tired, have hollow pits in my eye sockets, am aching and chilled, have had a lot of stomach upset and gas (not quite the runs).

The on-call nephrologists called—because Lynda's platelets are low, and he wants to avoid the use of heparin, they're going to try daily dialysis but take smaller steps. Her blood pressure has stabilized without dopamine, and she's slightly interactive today—though not communicative. Open eyes, says a visiting friend.

…She is apparently pretty agitated today, moving around and gurgling. The doctor called—a pulmonologist was called in to consider a ventilator, but his observation is that she is confused more than anything else, and her liver function and ammonia are out of whack. He is going to give her lactulose and feed her something that's nutritional but doesn't put a load on the liver to synthesize.

He was asking just how aggressively we wanted to pursue a ventilator etc. if that became necessary, but he basically answered his own question with how well she was doing *so* recently, and having 2 boys at home, etc.

My head hurts.

Our friend is being a real champ—seeing Lynda every couple hours at visiting hours and reporting to me. I can't do it any more—I'm burned out.

◆   ◆   ◆

E-mail—Tuesday, June 19th, 2001.
Subject: Lynda Status—Day 445

Lynda was transferred to intensive care over the weekend.

Thursday the dialysis procedure was too much for her, and her blood pressure took a big dip. She recovered from that, but then by Sunday she was septic again and confused, causing again decreased blood pressure—they had to put her on medication to keep it up and moved her to ICU. They've got her off that medication now, but have put her on a ventilator and sucked a bunch of gunk out of her lungs—she is obviously resting more easily now.

Every day, each new doctor, we get a slightly different story—kidney, lungs, liver, heart, fluid pressure, blood infection. Bottom line, she's a mess, and they're not sure what to do about it.

Thanks for all the prayers.

-GERALD

E-mail—Thursday, June 21st, 2001.

Subject: Lynda Status—Day 447

Yesterday they went in and cleaned out an abscess they had found in Lynda's liver. They removed about 200cc (almost a cup full) of infected material. If this sheltered reservoir of bacteria was responsible for re-seeding her blood infection, despite use of antibiotics, perhaps cleaning it out will open the door for forward progress from here.

Let's hope!

-GERALD

E-mail—Friday, June 22nd, 2001.

Subject: Lynda Status—Day 448

When I arrived to visit her today, Lynda saw me, decided it was time to go, and tried to get out of bed. We had to disappoint her—she was tied down a dozen ways (IV, blood pressure cuff, ventilator, feeding tube, catheter, oxygen monitor, drain for her abscess, EKG leads...), but she was ready. Actually, I couldn't get much more out of her that visit, but hey! this is progress!

Obviously cleaning out the abscess has removed a big hurdle to her getting better. The concern now is that if bacteria is collecting at sites in her liver, the stents (mesh tubes) she has holding open her bile duct really need to be changed out, and they can only do it at the transplant center. So, the wheels are now in motion to send her up over the mountain again—probably during the beginning portion of the week if not sooner.

I'm thinking I'll follow a few days later with the boys, hoping to visit and maybe bring her home end of the 4th of July week...Here's hoping!

-GERALD

Saturday, June 23, 2001

Dear Lynda,

As I write this you are starting to come up out of a period of unconsciousness. I am writing for the time when you can look back and try to understand.

They cleaned the big abscess out of your liver Wednesday evening (day 17 of this hospitalization) and you've been doing much better *but* if bacteria is collecting in your liver, the stents in your bile duct need to be changed out too, and that means back to the Transplant Center. They are likely to fly you over the mountain later today, or perhaps tomorrow. Hopefully, with these hurdles out of your way, you'll be able to recover from your very puzzling complex of problems. Frankly, we'd about given up on you until they found the abscess, which explained a lot.

Of course no one can predict how long it will be for you to recover enough to come home. It could be smooth sailing from here, but the road is still long.

I don't see any way you'll be coming home this coming week. In addition, several projects at work are coming to a head this week, projects we've been working on months and years. In short I need to stay here with the boys for this week.

If you're doing well and can come home, or at the very least are in a condition to visit with the boys, the following week has 4th of July on Wednesday, and we ought to be able to arrange to visit a whole or half a week or even take you home around then.

Of course I'll be there to get you whenever you are ready. (I know your heart and mind are ready. About the only thing you could do when I visited yesterday was to try to get out of bed to go the minute you saw me!)

We're still on for the beach trip July 21st. You've got that long—your presence is required at Ocean Isle. There are fish, birds, waves, boats, turtles, and little boys all requiring your observation.

We love you very much, can't wait to have you back. Everybody is asking about you and wants me to pass on their love to you. The boys especially miss you.

We'll see you soon!

Yours always,

   -GERALD

p.s. The pocket VCO (Voice Carry Over phone adaptor) should be in your baggage!

E-mail—Monday, June 25th, 2001.

Subject: Lynda Status—Day 451

Not much change over the weekend. Lynda will go to the transplant center the minute (or rather the day) they get an ICU bed available. She will go by air ambulance since she is still on the ventilator etc. She's conscious and restless, but not up to reading or writing levels of communication.

-GERALD.

Journal Entry, Tuesday, June 26

Because bacteria is collecting in her liver, they decided they really need to change out Lynda's stents, so she's on the waiting list to get a bed at the transplant center—and has been since last Friday.

She's been on a ventilator all this time but now is awake enough to be agitated and uncomfortable. She can't talk, hear, or write. She did manage to use a bed pan. Very upset another time when she made a mess and had to be cleaned.

Our friend says that when she told Lynda that I was with the boys, she cried.

This is bad enough on us, not knowing what is going to happen. This has to be horrible for Lynda.

◆   ◆   ◆

E-mail—Thursday, June 28th, 2001.
Subject: Lynda Status—Day 454

Lynda is doing better—off the ventilator, some improvement in her labs.

She is at that stage where her recent vivid dreams are more real than reality, and she mumbles quite sincerely about all kinds of wild things that she's sure happened. She won't accept that she needs to be there and was trying every way she could to get me to take her home—*right now;* they've had to restrain her so that she wouldn't pull out her tubes and fall on her face trying to get out of bed.

Ironically, her improvement has probably reduced her priority for an ICU bed at the transplant center, which is a rare commodity these days. Perhaps the proposed stent change was no more than precautionary—she is getting better, though slowly. She's still on the list and could move any day—or not. Stay tuned.

Thanks for all the support.

-GERALD

Journal Entry, Sunday, July 1

Last Thursday morning I visited, and she was off the respirator, speaking clearly but softly—hard to understand. She was clearly psychotic—living her dreams and asking questions about ridiculous stuff.

She was restrained because she was trying to pull off her leads and leave.

Saturday the nurse called—she was having a real good day, was NOT restrained, and was looking to call via the VCO phone adaptor. Was asking for me to visit.

So today I dropped the boys in the waiting room (with promises to take 'em to the Sword and the Stone if they were good) and went in to visit.

She was very weak. She opened her eyes a few times before trying to talk and trying to write, but I couldn't understand. Something about finding a woman in Wal-mart and was I going to divorce her. Obviously back in dream world.

They were giving her Flagyl—obviously no allergic reaction. Her abscess was still 10 cm, and they had put in a larger drain and were irrigating it. Not real clear whether CT scan had detected a leak as nurse had suggested from technician comments the night before. Blood count low—going to transfuse her. Albumin low. Good news was she's peeing more, and they plan to put off dialysis.

◆   ◆   ◆

E-mail—Monday, July 2nd, 2001.
Subject: Lynda Status—Day 458

Lynda is heading to the transplant center today, apparently by ground ambulance. She's had good days and bad days mentally—she is still fighting infections, and they are still hunting for sources. Hopefully the transplant center Docs will be able to clean out some nooks and crannies in her liver that haven't been accessible to date. They've put a larger drain in her abscess—it isn't just going away on its own.

-GERALD

Journal Entry, July 10

Here I am in the NC Botanical Gardens, having just fled from Lynda's hospital room. Yesterday was an up tick, today she's drowning in her own fluids.

I think I've figured out one of the paradoxes of modern medicine—the seeming senseless prolonging of life without much hope.

Before the transplant, they had to wait until having surgery was a better choice medically than leaving things be. In other words, Lynda had to suffer enough to *want* to have the transplant, grim and gruesome as a transplant might be. And indeed Lynda shifted from fearing it to hoping fervently it would happen in time. That attitude probably made all the difference when the time came, in terms of our preparation and her ability to face the operating room bravely, concentrating her energies on the fight.

I see a similar thing happening with the dying process. I've given up on Lynda's chances over and over again as her prognosis has shifted around. I see experts keep her body going, but even if she pulls through this round of hospitalizations, I know this entire series of events could recur as a result of a simple stomach flu. She will be back in the hospital again and again, and the fear of doctors will be greater each time, and she will be sicker and sicker each time. IF she doesn't die here and now at the transplant center, it will be sooner or later in some hospital somewhere, with tubes stuck in her…

My emotional attitude about her dying has evolved along a similar route to the progression of her own emotional attitude pre-surgery. I started out unwilling to face it, then moved to fearing it, then dealing with it as a possibility to be prepared for. Now as the probabilities arise, I am yanked back and forth between my "what if" plans—which I emotionally am trying to make seem good to ease my pain—and on the other hand the prospect of seeing Lynda go through months or years of agony and frustration with her illnesses, her disabilities, the *mis-match* of her former dreams and her current dark reality. I see myself sucked right along out of my sense of duty to her and responsibility for the kids—the desire to save our boys' Mom and to do right by my partner (buried somewhere in this emotional train-wreck).

By prolonging the dying process, those of us still here have time to see the alternatives and see that perhaps death is a better choice. NO—not choice, it is never *my* choice—maybe hers. Say a better alternative. I see Lynda choking on her own phlegm. She often can't clear it herself, so they come in every so often and stick a tube down her throat to suck it up. The idea is to get it down deep enough to do some good without making her throw up. They tried to put a tube through her nose for suction, and the result was a quart waste collector full of bloody spittle but still no tube in place.

Because she can't swallow, they had to stop feeding her via the nose tube—if she regurgitated it, she could choke to death.

And of course she hates to be suctioned—she bites the tube and resists. Her lips and teeth are still bloody from the night's adventures.

Right after being suctioned she can talk well—said "It was not a very sophisticated solution but it would do." The three things she talked about were 1) her choking on phlegm, and the clearing thereof, 2) being hungry (sausage and bacon was the request yesterday, wanted us to go out for a salad today), and 3) wanting to be hugged and cuddled—wanted me to climb in bed with her. Of course there is nothing I can do to deliver her from any of these miseries. I can only take so much of that and have to flee—think about boys—revert to my own childhood pastimes in search of comfort. Over-eat to answer that empty feeling inside, then fight acid reflux all night instead of sleep.

Lynda is in hell, and I'm having my nose rubbed in it. Yes, I can see that she would be better off. In my agony I wish for resolution—not really for death since life would be better, but limbo and agony forever is clearly worse than either. Especially for someone with a lifetime fear of doctors.

So is that the role of modern medicine? In a society where we don't see death up close and personal any more—don't see much suffering of the human condition—we must see how intensely bad it can be, before death seems an acceptable alternative.

Personally I've always felt that no agony is too great to endure if it meant one more chance to be an effective person in the world, fighting for whatever values you hold dearest. I could see sacrificing yourself for some greater glory, but never giving up to avoid a temporary evil. All through this, I've wished I could make Lynda see that to give her more strength. Now that faith in me is undermined as I see the effectiveness of that brief time later undercut by the psychosis of having suffered, and the waves of destruction and dysfunction you leave behind in the people around you. How can you ever judge and balance things like that? Being with Lynda has made me think about it. Maybe it's a question with no answers—"Ya pays yer nickel and ya takes yer chances."

I was puzzled by certain nurses' attitudes, seemingly offended that I was not by Lynda's side at the local hospital every minute. They were assuaged by our friend telling them I had kids to think about and care for. Perhaps they understood that the only point of all this modern medicine, prolonging of agony, was to teach me, the loving care giver, that death was a better alternative. My not being there made the agony pointless and cast them in the roll of senseless torturer. I guess I could see how they would resent that.

I've certainly come to the point that I could deal with any outcome. My challenge now is to deal with the time of uncertainty. Looking to the boys, they have been living with the possible loss of the Mom for some time. Even the youngest has asked me whether she's coming back this time and gotten unusually huggy. What can I do to ease their transition? They seem to have thrown themselves into collecting Warhammers (Science Fiction/Fantasy versions of tin soldiers—with battle rules and everything). I've tried to be a part of that for them.

What am I doing here at the transplant center, hundreds of miles from home and the boys? Few out in the world need the roller-coaster updates. I don't think I'm helping Lynda much—I can't give her what she needs. She shows more gratitude to the guy who suctioned her than to me. Her life has really spiraled down to the day to day minutia.

I need to take this time to build back my strength, to work out a plan for the uncertainty of a likely return to home without Lynda and no sign of resolution. How do I plan for the family while life hangs on tenterhooks for weeks, months, or years. I don't think I can have faith that a Lynda "recovered" is robust enough, steady enough, dependable enough, to build a future around. What to do, what to do…?

The boys need more stable figures in their life. The roles of Auntie, the CNA, and the families we've befriended become very important.

◆   ◆   ◆

Journal Entry, Friday the 13th, July 2001.

Had some good long discussions with two doctors in the last two days, one from Internal Medicine and the other her liver specialist.

The stuff in her lungs is staph. Two theories compete—either the stomach flu caused dehydration which caused pneumonia, which crossed into her blood stream, then moved to create the abscess in her liver, *or*, the abscess had been there all along, possibly related to the bile duct stents, and simply served as a source for the staph when conditions were just right. In support of this latter theory, her liver function remains good despite the abscess and despite the fact that it does not just drain and collapse down. The suggestion is that the main site of infection is the bile duct stents (possibly blocked), and that it is draining *into* the abscess.

I hoped to distinguish between these since one suggests a specific cause which we could FIX and never have happen again. The other suggest it "just happened" and could happen again at any time. The endoscopy might tell the story if it proved or disproved a physical link between the bile duct and the abscess—with tremendous implications for the years ahead. The Internist basically said that when bad things like this start happening, they tend to keep on happening. The liver specialist said don't expect the endoscopy to be very diagnostic—we may never be able to distinguish between the two cases but in a sense it didn't matter because indeed her metabolism *is* fragile. She is immuno suppressed, she has limited kidney capacity so is vulnerable to dehydration, and she is colonized by all kinds of nasty, antibiotic resistant bugs (VRE, MRSA, and ARSA) that we can never get rid of completely and will always be there waiting for an opportunity.

The liver specialist has seen patients have trouble for a year then "fly", but he is disappointed in Lynda's outcome and prone to be pessimistic.

Bottom line—the only thing we can count on is if she gets out of this one without something worse taking her away, she will still have this fragile metabolism and so get sucked back into the hospital regularly until one such visit finally finishes her off.

Based on this, I resolved to push forward on the plan to introduce more stable and permanent adult influences into our family, because one firm leg on the stool of their emotional support is simply not enough. Transition will be very problematic, I need to find someone whose role can change gradually as the situation changes, and willing to string along with that understanding.

Auntie has first claim if she wants it, but then she'd be leaving career, family, and community ties behind her. Plus, she never chose to raise a family of her own before this. I expect she will want to remain a "Mary Poppins" figure who drops in when most needed, then goes her own way—rather than wading into the chaos of family like a "Maria Von Trapp". I've put the question to her and she needs time to think about it.

The other obvious possible supplemental mom for my boys would be the certified nursing assistant (CNA) that has taken care of Lynda in the home. She has become very involved with our kids these nearly two years, and she would be sorely missed by them if she were to be displaced and moved on. She has kids of her own and would probably welcome the relief from her very deep financial hole. I don't know how she'd feel about this on a personal level. She always seems to have a man on a string and may not want to commit to such an uncertain relationship with myself and Lynda.

Both Auntie and the CNA have been good partners to work with, in different situations, during this time. Others of similar quality would be very hard to find.

But on to today's plans: The long awaited ERCP (procedure to run tubes down her esophagus and dilate her bile duct from below), the reason for a transfer to the transplant center, much delayed first by no bed, for the transfer, then by her infectious condition, then by scheduling—the key, perhaps to understanding Lynda's future.

They started giving her anesthesia, saw that she didn't have enough oxygen in her blood to deal with full anesthesia, and aborted the procedure. Maybe next week.

What a Catch 22—she remains sick, possibly because of the bile duct, but as long as she stays sick, they can't work on her bile duct. We're back to hoping she'll get better, when weeks of vancomycin and days of draining her abscess have not produced that result. This was termed an "optional" procedure by the endos-copy specialist, but I see this as a major set-back to hopes of recovery.

I'll visit again this afternoon, then it'll be too late to drive, so I'll stick to my plan to leave Saturday morning. Auntie says she might make it down Thursday, for a long weekend.

I don't know how much good my visiting does. Half the time she spends try-ing to convince me to smuggle either her out, or food in—and to make arrange-ments for an RN to take care of her at the house (two so they can do shifts). The other half of the time she's problem-solving our domestic situation which in some ways is pure fantasy but in other ways not. She recognizes that she won't be there forever for the boys and is looking to live by the transplant center to be closer to support groups and health care. She is asking for a contractor we know back home to do some remodeling work so that she has a modest apartment to live in and here we get confused on geography between home and here.

Lynda's fantasy is that I've *already* linked up with some woman, that we are negotiating custody of the children, and keeps asking about my "in-laws". She asks if I call this woman girlfriend—or wife now? I deny it and ask who can help me with the boys, and then she points to the CNA. Clearly not the same person in her mind.

It's spooky though, that for all her delirium and wrong facts, she has quite a grip on what she thinks *ought to be*. Her fearful assumption is that she has to be <u>displaced</u> to make room for a new mother for the boys, and she is trying to nego-tiate herself a modest but comfortable spot to finish out her days.

Perhaps I'm naïve or just eccentric, but I want the boys to have both—their own mother as long as they can *plus* a more stable maternal figure that they can rely upon to be there with them for the long haul. I think it can be done. A part-nership for the purpose of providing for children need not include a personal relationship between me and all the people emotionally important to my chil-dren. I intend to find a way.

Again, the need to put my own personal needs and desires on hold for my pri-mary goal—the kids. I'm ready to do or sacrifice what I must to help them develop into emotionally stable adults they could be—if only…

They have such potential. What a tragic waste if they were left to drift. Stay with the vision….

…Lynda's pulse wandered around from low 40's to high 80's afternoon and evening—possibly as a result of anesthesia. Was not wakeful in evening when I visited.

◆   ◆   ◆

Journal Entry, Saturday, July 14th, 2001.

My goodbye. They had her restrained by feet as well as hands since she was swinging her legs over the rail to go. She was quite psychotic, upset that I hadn't brought a lawyer, discussing need for a big-name lawyer, getting 5-8 of us to zip off together to some secret place overseas where we'd be safe, and some 250 to 350 million dollars being at stake. I could choose anyone I wanted to take with us. I was instructed *not* to return without a lawyer and a legal solution to our problems.

◆   ◆   ◆

E-mail—Monday, July 16th, 2001.
Subject: Lynda Status—Day 472

I just spent a week with Lynda at the transplant center. Things could be better, could be worse. Basically they're treating symptoms and trying to keep her comfortable, but are having trouble getting at the root causes. Lynda's pneumonia and blood infections are somewhat better, and her organs are all doing their jobs. However, the (10 cm) abscess in her liver is *not* going away despite all the antibiotics they're pumping through her. One procedure they wanted to do had to be aborted because she couldn't take the anesthesia. She's alert but living in fantasy land—plotting her daring escape to some overseas international safe haven from which she would pursue further high-tech spy-thriller intrigues—they've had to take some extreme measures to keep her from falling on her face.

Looks like the boys will be in school again before she's home—best case.

-GERALD

Journal Entry, July 21, 2001

Auntie is down there—says Lynda was back to gargling on her own fluids. Yesterday morning they couldn't rouse her and discovered her CO_2 levels had climbed (even though O_2 was good), because she was not breathing deep enough. They intubated her and sent her to ICU. Prevailing theory is that she was not clearing the anti-depressant medicine fast enough, and it built up too high—sedation effect—probably nutritional related as the liver produces the proteins/enzymes that break this stuff down—but the liver seems okay. They hope to get her off ventilator again in a couple of days. Of course it is possible something else is going on like the pneumonia advancing. She was alert this morning but needed assistance breathing.

◆   ◆   ◆

E-mail—Monday, July 23rd, 2001.
Subject: Lynda Status—Day 479
    The roller coaster took a couple bounces this weekend. Friday they put Lynda back on a ventilator. The theory was a sedation effect from a medication they were giving her, which built up higher than expected. Her reduced nutrition slowed down the liver's metabolizing of the drug, so it cleared slower than expected. They've been saying it would take a day or two to clear the CO_2 out of her bloodstream and getting her breathing 100% on her own again, but they've been saying that for three days now. They keep working on draining the abscess—still have not changed out the stents in her bile duct (the reason I thought we went to the transplant center), but they're thinking now that there really isn't a connection.
    Stay tuned, and keep praying.
    Thanks,
    -GERALD

E-mail—Monday, July 23rd, 2001.
To: Friend
Subject: RE: Comments on Lynda Status—Day 479
    What I can't imagine is if Lynda gets home—IF—there is nothing to stop this from happening as the aftermath to annual flu (yes she had shots) again, and again. You know what it's like with kids. Her metabolism just isn't up to it, and she's colonized by all these nasty bugs. So, she has every reason to expect to spend 3 months out of every year, for the rest of her life, being tortured in the hospital. No notice, no way to plan ahead. How would/will she cope with *that*?
    -GERALD

Journal Entry, July 25.

Yesterday finally pulled the stents out of her bile duct. No communication with the abscess found. They also did a lot of work on her abscess drain—increasing the diameter of the tubing. "A lot of necrotic tissue" plugging the drain, using

TPA to dissolve clots and help it drain. Still on the ventilator for a few more days at least.

♦   ♦   ♦

E-mail—Wednesday, July 25th, 2001.
Subject: Lynda Status—Day 481.

They finally pulled the stents out of Lynda's bile duct. This is fine now, and in no way connected to the liver abscess, which they are still trying to clear up. They keep on working the drain in the abscess and have it draining again. Chest x-rays are reportedly better, so they're hoping to start moving towards getting rid of the ventilator.

-GERALD

Journal Entry, July 27.

EXTUBATED!

♦   ♦   ♦

E-mail—Friday, July 27th, 20001.
Subject: Lynda Status—Day 483.

Just got word that they took Lynda off the ventilator. Progress! Her drain is draining. Step by step…

-GERALD

E-mail—Tuesday, July 31st, 2001.
To: Lynda's Brother

Lynda was moved back to the step-down unit now that she's off the ventilator (is on oxygen mask). Her mental status comes and goes—she's talking some. The optimistic doctors are saying she'll be here at *least* a week more but might go back to a regular room in that time frame. They're asking about the level of care she'd get here and thinking about rehab plans. They've drained lots of fluid out of her abscess, but the question is—is it closing up and healing? They keep running scans, but I'm not getting the data so don't know. They've cultured some of the gunk and decided to switch to a penicillin cousin this week—were planning to "desensitize" her as she is allergic to penicillin. Don't ask me, I don't know how they do that.

No I've not called your folks often recently—nothing to report really.

-GERALD

E-mail—Thursday, August 2nd, 2001.
Subject: Lynda Status—Day 489.

Lynda continues to improve mental status which is a good sign of progress on the over-all staph infection. She's no longer restrained for her safety and is operating the TV remote, being set up in a chair, etc. They're doing swallowing studies to see if she can get back on solid food. She hasn't tried using her VCO phone adapter yet, but it can't be too much longer. They "desensitized" her to a cousin of penicillin (to which she is allergic) that is better targeted at the bug in her liver abscess, and they are doing lots of monitoring to see whether the abscess is getting better. Looks like she'll be making it home after all—thanks for all the prayers and good thoughts!

-GERALD

E-mail—Monday, August 6th, 2001.
Subject: Lynda Status—Day 493.

Well, Lynda is back in the ICU. They tried letting her have soft foods, but it seems a noticeable portion ended up in her lungs. At any rate her x-rays show a big increase in the gunk in her lungs, and she's had more trouble breathing. They are watching her closely, and considering whether they need to intubate her for the ventilator again. They say it will be at least a couple weeks before they'd try her on semi-solid foods again, and can't keep the tube in her nose indefinitely—they are very close to putting a feeding tube directly into her stomach.

Still a rocky road…

-GERALD

Journal Entry, August 7.

She progressed up to the point of trying semi-solid foods and was pretty alert—still fantasizing about what was going on in her absence and not able to use the pocket VCO. The food was a mistake, as it appeared in the chest X-rays in her right lung. Sunday they called saying she was going back to ICU because her breathing was poor. Monday they told me she got intubated again before she even got to the ICU. Her abscess has shrunk—but only from 10.5 by 7.5 down to 8.5 by 7.5 centimeters, and it should be GONE before they remove the drain.

As I see it, they've been trying to kill this staph (MRSA or Methicillin Resistant Staph Aureus) in her lungs for over 2 months now. Getting food into her lungs can only have set her back, and strengthen the MRSA infection. Overnight intubation was more abrupt than the Doc on Sunday indicated. It is advancing alarmingly.

◆   ◆   ◆

Journal Entry, Saturday, August 11.

On Thursday Lynda underwent a tracheostomy and had a tube placed directly into her treachea for improved breathing. It supposedly went well though continued oozing of blood delayed the second thing they wanted to do—the stomach feeding tube. Drove down Friday late afternoon and arrived coincident with a major cloudburst and pyrotechnic thunder storm. Lynda woke up for a head rub. Was very weak but had enough fight to kick off the sheet 67%. She recognized me and mouthed "I love you" and "Help me," but I couldn't understand much except that she wanted to get up. She was obviously miserable and the nurse came in and gave her morphine and Atovan to knock her out.

...Spoke with the ICU doctor. He says the pneumonia is "not that bad"—effects of aspirating food could have been ten times worse. Problem is she is too weak to do her own breathing and will probably be on and off the ventilator until she gets her strength back—which may not be until she heals the abscess. And of course it has taken 2 months to drop it 2 centimeters—does this mean 8 more to go!? They keep culturing it to monitor whether they're doing the right thing to kill the bacteria and are trying things like TPA.

...She begs me to help her, but of course there is nothing I can do. This just tears me up. They haven't fed her in days due to complications and she's hungry.

◆   ◆   ◆

E-Mail—Wednesday, August 15th, 2001.
Subject: Lynda Status—Day 502.

With the trachea tube now it place, they can easily move Lynda on and off the ventilator depending on her strength & sedatives given. This also gives her about 10% more breathing capacity since it bypasses that much dead space.

Her pneumonia really isn't that bad, they assure me, could have been 10x worse after aspirating food. Problem is she's just too weak to do all her own breathing and probably will stay that way until they can heal up the big abscess in her liver. Progress on that front is very spotty, but that's where the action (or inaction) is. We've passed the 10 week point this visit and the abscess has only dropped from 10.5 to 8.5 cm. We're in for a long haul.

They are going to place a feeding tube directly through the wall of her stomach today, so they can feed her and build up some strength without the risk of it getting into her lungs.

She had some fairly lucid moments when I visited this weekend. Sedation is merciful though, as she can't talk or hear and is restrained to avoid pulling out tubes.

-GERALD

E-Mail—Monday, August 20th, 2001.
Subject: Lynda Status—Day 507

Lynda seems to be responding well to the direct tube feed to the stomach. The trachea tube is helping on the breathing—they are spending a lot of time on just room air. Doing stuff like sitting in chairs again, OT, PT, etc. They are talking about moving her down to a regular hospital room in the next few days. No data on how much or even whether that abscess is shrinking—they've had to reposition the drains again.

Definitely on an upswing…

-GERALD

Journal Entry, Sunday, August 26.

Twelve weeks! She's been out of ICU for a week now—feeding tube through stomach wall obviously did her good. Can't go too fast though, due to pain. She's been lethargic and moderately communicative. Put her back on Haldol for psychosis. Continuing to claim the abscess is shrinking but very slowly. Trachea is on humidified room air only. Has yet to rally enough to punch keys on a phone. Auntie is going down for 5 days labor day weekend.

◆   ◆   ◆

Journal Entry, August 30.

Back on "solid" foods again. Doctors are cautiously optimistic based on her condition and labs, but can offer only vague platitudes about progress with the abscess.

◆   ◆   ◆

E-mail—Tuesday, September 4th, 2001.
Subject: Lynda Status—Day 522

Things are definitely looking up! They are working towards moving Lynda to the local Rehab hospital by the end of this week! A host of things could still delay this, but the end is in sight!

The drain from Lynda's liver has been removed, and the abscess has progressed to "another phase of care"—she'll be on I.V. antibiotics for months I think. She still has the trachea tube and feeding tube, but she's eating again and talking with the valve on the trachea—I'm sure we'll be getting rid of these tubes soon. Best of all, she is perking up and more herself again—she was able to operate the phone adaptor for the deaf and call a number of people this weekend. She has even taken an outdoor trip in the wheel chair.

Thanks for all the prayers!

-GERALD

E-mail—Tuesday, September 11th, 2001.
Subject: Lynda Status—Day 529

A bright spot on this dark day—

Lynda moved to the local Rehab hospital yesterday. She made the trip well and is in very high spirits. She's weak and thin as a toothpick but is full of energy and seems herself again. Perhaps she can make it to the house in a week or so.

Visiting hours are 4-9 M-F, 1-8 Sat, 8-8 Sun. She'll be busy with PT etc. most of the rest of the time. You can phone to the front desk—they may be moving her around, so I hesitate to give a room number.

-GERALD

E-mail—Wednesday, September 12th, 2001.
Subject: Lynda Status—Day 530

Lynda's coming home Friday at noon. They say she's using a walker.
-GERALD

Journal Entry, Friday, September 14th, 2001.

Lynda came back to the local Rehab hospital on Monday. She saw the traumatic events of September 11 on TV and had them call me and ask if I needed to pull the kids out of school. She is walking with the walker and doing so well they agreed to let her go home Friday. She's getting two IV antibiotics daily for 2-3 weeks and Epogen shots. Cancelled at the last minute due to her nausea. The CNA noticed poor appetite the day before and signs of confusion today. We'll see if she makes it home this weekend.

❖   ❖   ❖

E-mail—Monday, September 17th, 2001.
Subject: Lynda Status—Day 537 (Note: I miss counted here, nobody noticed).

Change in plans...Lynda is still at the Rehab hospital because she has C. Difficile in her gut again (this is the bug that moves in when antibiotics kill everything else). This has to get under control before we can care for her at home. Hopefully we can get her home this week, but we're taking it day by day....

-GERALD

E-mail—Wednesday, September 19th, 2001
Subject: Lynda Status—Day 539

Lynda is actually home now, for real! Got through the first night with no problems. She is standing and walking but needs help with balance. Will be close to home for awhile, as she's getting IV's through home health 8am and 8pm. Finally got a figure on her "residual abscess"—it has dropped from the original 10.5 cm to "only" 5.5 centimeters (in two months of care). I guess she stays on the IV antibiotics until it's gone....

From here on out, figure no news is good news. Thanks for hanging with us...

-GERALD

21

Finding Peace

	Winter	Spring	Summer	Fall
1988	(2) Engagement	(3) Wedding		
1989	(13) Reflections on Adoption			(4) Adoption
90-95	(4) Raising our Children			
1996			(5) Swelling	(1) Christmas
1997	(5) Diuretics	(5) Dehydrated	(5) Encephalop-athy	(5) Encephalop-athy
1998	(5) Encephalopa-thy	(5) Encephalopa-thy	(5) On the List	(6) Holding to Family
1999	(6) Holding to Family	(7) Big Crash, Shunt	(8) Dominos Falling	(9) Live Donor?
2000	(9) Aborted Hopes	(10) Transplant (11) Closing Up (12) Lingering	(13) Beacon (14) Long Dis-tance	(14) Rehab (15) Hearing Loss (16) Home Care
2001	(16) Bile Drains	(17) Reflec-tions—Me (18) & on the Kids (19) Insurance	(20) Abscess	**(21) Finding Peace**

I have finally found a measure of peace, a place of calm after this long journey. How can this be? Nothing has changed outwardly. Lynda is returning from 14 weeks in hospital—our workload will go up again soon, and she is again at high risk for a fall, which will require our 24 hour-a-day attention. The medical glitches continue too; she has C. Difficile again, so her return home is delayed a few more days. We have every reason to believe Lynda is very fragile and will continue to pop in and out of the hospital regularly for the rest of her life until one of these episodes gets her. Our counselor tells me that her day-to-day survival probability is less than that of many cancer patients she sees. In short, we're looking ahead to one of several bad endings with a lot of work and uncertainty ahead. Pretty grim—and yet I've gained a new perspective, thanks to our counselor.

Lynda and I were both independent sorts, and our marriage has somewhat of an "us against the world" alliance. This was a source of strength for me through the first four and a half years of her disease. I felt the duty and responsibility to help my partner through every problem, and I was able to rise to the occasion. The burden got too great for me to bear, though, and I was overwhelmed with despair at our situation. These last few months were killing me. Particularly the fact that Lynda was in denial over the seriousness of the situation really drove it home, adding insult to injury, underlining the fact that I really was all alone, without a partner, to bear the burden for us all.

Our counselor confirmed for me that Lynda no longer would have what it took to be a partner. She had had enough of a time last spring in trying to get Lynda outside her problems and to think about anyone else. With no end of torment in sight, she never would recover her ability to partner, and I would be fooling myself to think that she might. The counselor was amazed that I had held on, fighting for the both of us for this long, alone. She said that I *would* find support and comfort elsewhere. It would be very unhealthy for me to try to live the lie of stepping into Lynda's fantasy that things could be the same again.

Let's be clear here—I love Lynda, and I admire her courage and spunk, her ability to fight back. I still feel responsible for caring for her and supporting her—as a dependent now. But I lost my partner three years ago. I still want her to be there for my boys—they need their mom and need to see a happy ending. I want her to give everything she has left to the boys, not me.

What about Lynda, what did she need? If she wants to connect with people again and find some meaning in this, the final stages of her life, she has to stop living in this fantasy that things will return to normal, lose her gripping fear of death, and learn to accept her new role in life with grace and dignity. She needs to stop planning an unrealistic future, and instead set about tidying things up the way she wants them to be when she departs. How could I bring that about? No way on Earth, and the burden of that responsibility was what was killing me.

My peace came from realizing this, and letting it go. Not only was I not equipped to help, having had neither the life experience to help her face death, nor the tools by training, any attempt by me to push Lynda towards taking this role, would be taken by her as a rejection by me. What she needed from me was simple love and support. It was simply not my job to lead Lynda to and through this stage of her life. That would fall to our counselor, and other contacts that Lynda had yet to make.

For me it was time to rest and heal, to wait patiently for this phase to pass before trying to get on with my life. Where would I find another emotional partner? No way to know, but that was a problem for the distant future, not now. What would happen to the boys and how would it affect their lives? Not in my control, except to be there for them, help them keep their friends and community ties available, and keep myself healthy and alive for them. I could choose to beat my head against an unsolvable problem, or let things come in their own time; the unsolved problems of the future would be confronted later, not now. All I could do worrying about them now would be to give myself a fatal coronary.

I had given Lynda everything I could. Now was the time for *me* to heal.

22

Last Shake of the Roller Coaster

	Winter	Spring	Summer	Fall
1988	(2) Engagement	(3) Wedding		
1989	(13) Reflections on Adoption			(4) Adoption
90-95	(4) Raising our Children			
1996			(5) Swelling	(1) Christmas
1997	(5) Diuretics	(5) Dehydrated	(5) Encephalop-athy	(5) Encephalop-athy
1998	(5) Encephalopa-thy	(5) Encephalopa-thy	(5) On the List	(6) Holding to Family
1999	(6) Holding to Family	(7) Big Crash, Shunt	(8) Dominos Falling	(9) Live Donor?
2000	(9) Aborted Hopes	(10) Transplant (11) Closing Up (12) Lingering	(13) Beacon (14) Long Dis-tance	(14) Rehab (15) Hearing Loss (16) Home Care
2001	(16) Bile Drains	(17) Reflec-tions—Me (18) & on the Kids (19) Insurance	(20) Abscess	(21) Finding Peace **(22) Complica-tions**

Journal Entry, November 13.

Well, things proceeded about as expected—painfully.

The Epogen shots for anemia were turned down by Blue Cross, and would have been $1200, so they decide she didn't need it that bad.

Of course she came down with C. Dif pretty quick, so we went on oral Vanco for a month to try and be sure. A week off it, and she had C. Dif right back again—we're on a 2-week second regime—I'm skeptical that it will be enough. Later a Doctor told me she'd not have a chance to clear the C. Dif. until she was off the antibiotics.

We went back to the transplant center for a check-up and they said she was great. We didn't need to come back until March for routine annual checkup. She was climbing stairs and starting to talk about driving.

The abscess appears to have been sterile and we were almost to the point it had shrunk enough to dispense with the IV's.

Then, our next episode hit.

Last Wednesday or so she started with runs and vomiting—a lot of this going around. No fever right up through Friday, when the CNA had to call and call to try and get an appointment, which was set for Monday.

4:30 Friday she still had no fever. Three hours later it was up 3 degrees, and it spiked to at least 102°. I think we got a reading of 102 in her arm pit at one point too, which would be 103°, but I can't be sure with the flakey digital thermometer.

Sent the two boys two different directions for the night—the oldest was primed for a Scouting bike trip Saturday morning—and we headed for the ER.

By time we got in, the fever was gone. The ER Doc looked in her ears etc. and decided she had a virus, not flu, looked well hydrated, and sent us home with pain killer for sinusitis, Phenergan and Imodium for the runs and vomiting. Said if the fever came back we'd have to return for abdominal CT scan.

Saturday she ran a low-grade fever and started itching all over. We broke out the Benadryl, which didn't help much.

Sunday morning Lynda was acting punch-drunk. She couldn't play Rummy right with the boys and started telling our older boy about aliens. I came in and felt her forehead, and she thought we were playing the poker game where you put a card on your forehead, so started flipping over her Rummy cards and holding them to her forehead.

At this point I said, "get packed, we're going to the ER." Somewhere in there we noticed her eyes were very yellow and bulgy.

But then I got to thinking—this is less confused and more "tipsy silly". I questioned her about her self-dosage of Benedryl, and she was obviously confused; said she had one at 4:00 pm during the night.

So I got on gloves and went through the trash, trying to account for the number of Benedryls she had taken by looking for the little plastic bubbles they come in. I had to sort through bloody Kleenex from her nose bleeds and used ginger ale from her vomiting but ultimately counted 12 she'd taken since we got to bed 3:00 am Saturday. This was 11:00 am Sunday—best we could piece together was that she'd had six on Saturday, so perhaps she'd had six in a five hour span on Sunday morning where the normal dose was 1-2 every 4-6 hours. She was high on antihistamine, but was still itching so much she had ripped her shoulders to shreds with the bamboo back-scratcher.

I decided we'd wait 'till Monday and called off the ER visit.

Her tipsiness cleared but she was still a bit slow on Monday. Out in the sun her skin glowed neon yellow.

We signed the refinance papers on the house, knocking off two percentage points, and headed for the Doctor. (We saw the Nurse Practitioner at first, but she took one look and pulled in the family Doctor). The jaundice, the itching from the billirubin build-up, maybe even the spike of fever all sounded to me like a bile duct blockage—though we all feared it might be something worse.

The local Doc called the local liver specialist and the transplant center, trying to decide how to proceed. The liver specialist said, "admit her," but not where. The transplant center agreed with the local doctor that the special tests needed had to be run at the transplant center, so the plan was to drive down out of the mountains and go back there.

Lynda was of course horrified and protested vehemently. She cried about what this was doing to the family, but in the end we really had no choice.

We recovered the boys for the night, got them off to school with arrangements for their care, and headed back.

Four and one half hours drive, with me tearing up over what a mess life was these days, considering the prospect of doing all this over and over again for years to come. Resentful that I'm put in the position of being between two bad possible outcomes—that Lynda's passing away (not a good thing) was the only relief in sight.

We've been here two and a half hours now, and the ER Doc has looked at her—is ordering basic blood tests and going to pass her on to the liver Doctors.

I imagine—WHOOPS! They came for X-rays. I got to stand in a lead vest and signal her when to take deep breaths, while the technician was around the corner operating the machine.

I was saying—I imagine they will admit her tonight and I'll have to go find a hotel and dinner. Have no reservations this time but don't expect trouble. Only had two donuts for lunch, and a cookie and small pastry for breakfast—no snacking on the way over. Partly I'm excited at being down to 270 pounds—first time I've seen that weight since the transplant, but mostly I'm sick to my stomach of all this.

A piece of it is a solid feeling that I'm really alone here, and it's foolish to think I can find anyone who could be an emotional partner with me while I'm still married to Lynda, and of course walking away from it all would refute everything my life values are about. My two best (only) candidates clearly don't want the "job". Three years of emotional isolation and who know how many more ahead of me, at which point I'll have to deal with losing Lynda *and* traumatized boys, with nobody standing ready to help smooth the transition. So depressing with no way out.

My counselor tells me, none of my problems are urgent except for my own health—I've *got* to drop my blood pressure; 150/110 when I woke up this morning. I've got to step back and let time resolve what it will, stop butting my head against brick walls.

◆   ◆   ◆

Journal Entry, Thursday, November 15.

I'm sitting here Thursday morning while they do ERCP (endoscopy) to clear out Lynda's bile duct, which definitely needs it. However, there is more going on.

The ultrasound found that one of the three veins that drain the liver is totally blocked off with a clot, and that there is a narrowing in the right femoral artery.

There was no way to tell by ultrasound whether the clot was old, and whether the surrounding vasculature had rearranged to compensate, or whether it was new, in any way related to the jaundice, or even causing the bile duct build-up.

I think of her recent fall and hematoma that she tried to conceal from me on the previous Tuesday—earlier on the same day in which she had later announced her intentions to drive our oldest boy to the dance in the dark—first drive since leaving hospital and I gave her a piece of my mind. It was like she had something to prove, but she shouldn't be practicing needlessly with other lives at stake.

They wanted to do an MRI to get details on the clot; and maybe learn more about need for ERCP. They only have the enclosed MRI here, and she has freaked out over the claustrophobia in the past. They promised to knock her out for the study, and I went back to the hotel.

In the morning I learned that they had needed her awake to hold her breath etc. after all, so she had balked and made them cancel the study.

So now she's getting the ERCP, but this won't shed any light on the mystery of the role of the clot. A different Doc would decide about how to treat it, so it wasn't the ERCP Doctor's call, but sounds like they'd start a course of drugs here and get her stabilized before letting her go home. Sounds like we're into the weekend now. Auntie is coming to the house Wednesday—I sure hope we're home for Thanksgiving!

I've got a sick feeling in the pit of my stomach that everything is slipping away. I have to be here with Lynda, but I'm turning my back on family, friends, work, home maintenance, etc. All my fragile efforts to build up normal family life for the boys is blown away like a house of cards.

...1:00. The endoscopy went fine, in fact her ducts were in good shape. They pulled a very little bit of mucus out—no significant debris; in fact, not enough to explain her symptoms. Evidently the clot (or something else) is playing a more significant role than we realized.

◆   ◆   ◆

Journal Entry, Sunday, November 18th, 2001

The clot was in the veins that *drain* the liver, not arteries that feed it. A lot of testing later we established that it was not caused by any narrowing or obstruction to the flow. Rather, the *Primaxin* antibiotic she was on was probably to blame. It is of the penicillin family, and people have been known to develop this reaction to it. With the switch to a new cocktail (assisted by the roto-rooter job on her bile duct) her bilirubin is dropping. If it continues, we may get out of here on Monday and be home for Thanksgiving.

She woke up with a bit of sore throat, wheeze, and cough, and I thought "Oh no!" but it cleared quickly as she was upright. Naps lots, and tires easily. Tomorrow is the big day!

◆   ◆   ◆

E-mail—Wednesday, November 28th, 2001.
Subject: Lynda Status—Day 609.

Wanted to pass on an update of our most recent "adventure". About 2 weeks before Thanksgiving Lynda developed flu-like symptoms. A fluky high fever had us into the ER Friday night but it was gone by time we arrived, and they sent us home "on watch". That weekend she started turning yellow and itching like crazy—billirubin backing up to make jaundice. By Tuesday we were back to the transplant center. It just took us a week this time to sort it all out. Her bile duct may have been slightly blocked but, more alarming, there was a clot in the veins that drain blood from the liver. This was likely caused by a reaction to one of the antibiotics she was taking for her abscess, which is much better but not quite gone. Anyway we made it home for Thanksgiving, and Lynda is now home enjoying the peace and quiet while coping with the "joys" of anticoagulants and, it seems, another round of C. Difficile infection in her gut. All in all though, she's happy to be home again!

-GERALD

Journal Entry, Monday, December 3rd, 2001

Well, the discharge was complex enough that we didn't get to go until Tuesday, but we *did* make it home for Thanksgiving, which we ate at the home of our family friends, joined by Auntie.

They stopped all the IV's and pulled out her pic line. Cipro was prescribed as the usual post-surgical prophylactic, though the local infectious disease Doc has confused the question regarding possibly continuing it awhile.

The anticoagulants are the big new thing. The Coumadin pills take time to build up in the blood stream—they'll take weekly blood levels to adjust dosage. This sounds like we're in for a long haul.

In order to bridge the gap until the pills are at full strength, we're to give twice daily injections of "Lovenox" for a week. These apparently sting like the dickens, and Lynda jumps and jerks and pulls away as I try (with my lack of depth perception) to get the needle and all the medicine in *her*, not me. She's really ill about it and accuses me of enjoying doing this to her. I tell her she can do it herself if she wants, but no.

Since this is anticoagulant, you can't even rub the spot afterwards, or you create a bruise. Most of the shots raised big bumps and many bled. We had lots of bleeding problems—the most worrisome was the site on the side of her neck where they did the angiogram. The most trouble was a blood-draw site on her arm that soaked several pressure bandages by breaking open again several times over a couple days until finally the visiting RN's told us to *clamp* it for at least 10 minutes, more if needed, then ice it. Our CNA finally got it to stop. I expect we'll get more of this sort of action until they stop the anticoagulants—though the worst might have been the overlap of the tail-end of the shots with the increasingly effective pills.

The boys both arranged to be with friends this weekend, and even when at loose ends didn't care to help me start the Christmas cookie batches.

Lynda slept in my (our) bed upstairs again, the first time in awhile. I made her promise to read elsewhere so I could go to sleep in the dark, and she said I could turn on lights to get dressed in the morning. I gave her grief about making a big deal tucking the boys in (first time in a long while) making them 25 minutes late to bed. I told her if she wants to be a help, to do it before Lights Out. We were 10 minutes late leaving the house in the morning (so I was late to work).

It is a lot of work getting the boys going in the mornings—I'm using a pot lid and wooden spoon, clanging them until the boys get vertical. They're still very slow, and act as if they just don't get it. I know it's deeper, but I can't keep fighting, so I'm finding low blood pressure ways to cope. I'm down to 135/90 on waking up and 271 ½ pounds this morning—sustainably at a weight I hadn't seen since the transplant.

◆   ◆   ◆

E-mail—Wednesday, December 5th, 2001.
To: Liver Coordinator
Subject: Query—Lynda—Cipro
Perhaps you can help us sort out some confusion…We came home with two weeks of CIPRO [note: I was wrong, just one week], then were to go cold turkey, no antibiotics unless the local infectious disease doctor wanted more. Upon visiting him, he questioned her status with the Cipro and asked Lynda to keep on taking the Cipro while he contacted somebody at the transplant center. I'm not sure third hand whether he was unhappy with her taking it in the first place, or the fact that it was stopping (given continued presence of abscess).

Now, Lynda did not know that the first Cipro prescription had run out, so I'm not sure whether the doctor knew this. Here's the thing—he did not write another prescription last week, and is not going very fast on getting in touch with somebody down there. I had 5-6 more days from an older bottle that didn't get used when Lynda went into hospital, so, since he said "keep on taking it" we've been using that up. However, we run out Saturday noon.

Could you help facilitate this dialog between the local doctor and Lynda's GI doctor there? If we're supposed to keep Lynda on it, we need to get a prescription in to the Pharmacy by Saturday.

Thanks,
-GERALD

Journal Entry, Sunday, December 16, 2001

The CNA and I have been comparing notes—Lynda keeps throwing a mental disconnect at us from time to time. We found a stray puppy, black lab, which she and the CNA ended up taking to the Animal Shelter for us (it was sure to get a home just before Christmas like this). The next day, Lynda asked if the CNA had seen the new puppy, and wondered where it was?

Monday they put off a flu shot because Lynda had sniffles. Wednesday they went for it, and then she started having serious flu symptoms like runs and headaches. The CNA had 'em too, so we figured it was nothing really odd, especially a mild fever after a flu shot.

Friday she began to itch and turn yellow. The family Doc ordered a CMP (Comprehensive Metabolic Panel) to check bilirubin, and a stool sample for C. Dif. (her oral vanco was to run out in 1 more day). She was still on Cipro. Her temperature bounced around 100 and her diarrhea was uncontrollable—I got to mop the floor before she was convinced to put on a diaper. Terrible sinus headache and shallow breathing. At first I thought her speech was slurred, but then I realized she was getting dehydrated and holding her lips funny—losing the "L" sounds. The lip thing I'd seen before in hospital—might be metabolic too.

The on-call Nurse Practitioner was consulted—all the E.R. could do was prevent dehydration (which we could do up to a point ourselves) and take another blood sample (while we were still waiting for the results of the first round). We decided to hang on and wait for the test results already in the pipe.

I made new arrangements for Saturday for our youngest boy to get to his morning-long wrestling tournament in the neighboring state. I drove our older boy to rendezvous with his scout troop for an overnight camp, and dropped a stool sample off at the lab. I had planned to go with our youngest, but now Lynda needed close watching.

Today, Sunday, she seems to be better, fever down. Running dehumidifier in her room is helping too. Imodium was controlling the diarrhea. She's not getting any more yellow from jaundice, and she's eating and holding it down. Sleeping a *lot* and isn't communicating well—a bit out of it.

We'll see what the blood tests show Monday. Christmas vacation is hanging in the balance.

◆   ◆   ◆

Journal Entry, Monday, December 17, 2001

This morning she was very lethargic and answered most questions with "okay" (including multiple choice ones). She raised a feeble protest over going to the hospital—insisted on something other than PJ's—though it turned out her jeans wouldn't fit over her diaper.

They got her into a room at the local hospital fast, and got a rather alarming blood pressure of 84/46. She screamed bloody murder over the blood draw and IV placement (took 1 try each). 84/49. 88/49. 76/42 at 11:43. 81/43. They strung up an IV bag but that didn't do much, blood pressure still 85/43.

12:55 pressure was 82/43. Her creatinin is high at 5 (showing kidney distress) but so is her bilirubin. Her platelets are ¼ normal, which is not due to the Coumadin (anti-coagulant). Her liver is somewhat enlarged. She does not seem to be carrying excess fluid. No indication of infection, but that is possible.

12:58 pressure was 76/40. Her heartbeat is only 65 which apparently does *not* go with dehydration.

In other words, whatever is going on is her usual complicated multi-factor puzzle. She'll be here days.

Saw one blood pressure of 78/36 but mostly about 80/45.

◆   ◆   ◆

E-mail—Tuesday, December 18th, 2001.
Subject: Lynda Status—Day 629

Lynda's back in the hospital again. In a sense it's a continuation of this summer's problems—her abscess is growing again. The antibiotics that had been healing it up were discontinued when they caused the blocked veins just before Thanksgiving. We had hoped the abscess was sterile enough to finish healing, but even with Cipro in her system, it rebounded and is now back up to an 8 centimeter hole in her liver. The kidneys decided it was time to take a vacation at that point, and the subsequent toxin build-up affecting her mind was what sent us to the local hospital on Monday. They hope to get her kidneys going again with fluids and maybe dialysis, though her low blood pressure (80/45) may complicate that. They have her back on the original antibiotics again, but now have to balance the anticoagulants & platelets (abnormally low) so that she doesn't have vein clotting problems again. On the other hand she doesn't bleed too much when they try to drain the abscess. As usual, Lynda presents quite a puzzle. No way of knowing whether she'll make it home for Christmas—time will tell.

Thanks for all the prayers—we still need 'em!

-GERALD

Journal Entry, Thursday, December 20, 2001.

After 3 days on IV fluids Lynda is still not communicative. This supposedly would be enough to restart her kidneys and flush out the toxins. Last night she ripped out her IV's which the Nurse called confusion, though I'd call an escape attempt.

Lynda does have a gall stone in her bile duct (according to MRI), so endoscopy is going to be necessary. As a result, they're going to ship her back to the transplant center—today if possible.

Her abscess is back up to 8 centimeters and needs draining—they may initiate that here before transporting her.

She is making a little bit of very dark urine, so her kidneys are still *there*—significant hope of another rebound.

They say her numbers look generally better, but the unrealized hope of rational communication by now is disappointing. More so is the fact that there is *no way* she'll be home for Christmas. It took weeks this summer to drain the abscess enough to remove the drain, and they won't send her home leaking a resistant strain of staph out of her side.

◆   ◆   ◆

Journal Entry, Friday, December 21, 2001

Last evening they flew Lynda to the transplant center—I stayed up late enough to verify that Lynda did get in—was puzzled why her room was in Respiratory ICU (only available bed?)—and got to sleep about Midnight.

2:45 a.m. I got a call from the Doctor who wanted permission to put in a central line (neck) and an arterial blood gas monitor in her wrist. The Doc told me Lynda had been intubated sometime at the local hospital between when the transport arrived and when the loaded her on the plane. The chest X-ray they got on her arrival shows several white *patches* in her lungs indicating she probably has pneumonia again now. "Patches" sounds worse to me than the "fuzzy areas" described to me before, but perhaps it's just a matter of how one says it, and how I took it. I asked about time frame—pointing out that it took more than a month of draining this summer to get the abscess to a state they could let her go. The Doc said the respiratory situation was more acute, and that she'd be on the respirator for some time.

They called and got permission to start the drains as well, though no one has contacted me with any results—probably was routine.

The boys know she won't be home for Christmas—I'm doubting whether she'll even be home in January. We all wondered if she'd live through flu season—she may not even make it to then.

◆   ◆   ◆

E-mail—Friday, December 21ˢᵗ, 2001.
Subject: Lynda Status—Day 632

They flew Lynda over to the transplant center last evening. Why they put her in Respiratory Intensive Care was a mystery until I got the 2:45 am call from the doctor, asking permission to put in central & arterial blood lines. They had put her on a respirator just before putting her on the plane. At the transplant center her x-rays showed several white patches on her lungs, so she probably has pneumonia again now, to go with the rest of her collection. They are actually considering this more of an "acute" issue than the abscess in her liver. She will definitely *not* be making it home for Christmas—or any time soon. We'll see what the New Year brings....

-GERALD

Journal Entry—Saturday, December 22, 2001

Lynda is initiating her own breaths now (still intubated), the drain is draining well, she's making urine. Her "septic" profile seems to be resolving—sedation is being held off now, so she ought to start waking up. No word from the GI Docs regarding plans to go after that bile duct stone.

...I can't begin to describe how hard it is to sit here tonight wrapping presents for the boys "from Santa Claus"—alone. I can't give them what they really need and want; I've been trying for 5 years to bring their Mom home, and I'm losing the fight. But neither is she actually gone; I am not free to find a new partner to care for these guys—no one will take on these boys as their own while I am still married. And of course no one else could even approach being their Mom in their eyes while their "real" mom is still battling for her life in and out of the hospital. So I am condemned to moments like this, carrying an unbearable burden, wrapping futile little presents for the boys, alone in the dark, and crying my eyes out.

Christmas Eve

They extubated her. Not sure she has a bile stone, are concerned about imaging whether bile is getting from the duct into her abscess, which would explain why it has been so hard to heal.

Christmas Day.

She's talking to the nurse but saying things that don't make any sense. Back to her ICU psychosis phase. We send our message of love, and hope for the best.

◆   ◆   ◆

Journal Entry—Wednesday, December 26th, 2001.

They extubated her Christmas Eve. Christmas she was talking but not making any sense.

Today she has some lucid moments and some confusion.

To better understand the state of her bile duct and abscess, they did a 2-hour "hi-da-scan" and have another 4-hour one later today. Right now her bile is not reaching her gut and is all coming out the abscess drain. It is possible the abscess is pressing on the duct and blocking it off by pressure. We will learn more.

◆   ◆   ◆

Journal Entry—Thursday, December 27th, 2001.

Not much joy today. They confirmed that there is serious connection between the bile duct and the abscess. Some sort of surgery is going to be required, if they can figure out what to do at all. The respiratory folks have got her stabilized and are looking to transfer her out of ICU into a step-down unit under the direct care of the liver folks. Now that she's breathing on her own, they can start to consider surgical options. Expect the surgeons to digest the situation and recommend a course of action no sooner than beginning of next week.

Auntie is going down Friday to spend a 4-day weekend with Lynda.

◆   ◆   ◆

E-mail—Thursday, December 27th, 2001.
Subject: Lynda Status—Day 638.

Lynda was extubated on Christmas Eve—off the respirator and just on some oxygen supplement. In general her vital signs are stabilizing, though her mental state goes in and out of the dream world.

The concern right now is that there is definitely a connection between her bile duct and the abscess. All her bile is flowing through the abscess and out the drain, instead of into her gut to help her digest. This is not a trivial matter, and will probably require some sort of surgical intervention to repair, if that is possible. The anatomy in question is inside the liver and hard to get at—not sure what they can do with endoscopy. It's also not clear what bile would do to the ability of a suture to heal, for instance—it clearly has been part of the problem with the abscess cropping up.

They have been waiting for Lynda to stabilize and build back up strength to consider surgery. They will probably move her out of the care of the Respiratory folks in ICU and into the care of the GI folks in a step-down unit. Expect the surgeons to be deciding what they can do for her beginning of next week. We'll see what the New Year brings.

-GERALD

Journal Entry—New Year's Day, 2002.

Lynda has been quite lucid the last couple days. Auntie visited this weekend—Lynda told her she didn't know why she was still alive.

Basically they've stabilized all her metabolic balances but need to resolve the bile-duct/abscess issues.

With so much bile going to the drain, it is questionable whether she can eat, and they need to do things to restore the more than one liter she's losing daily. This is a big drain on her metabolism.

They need to repair the leak but in her weak condition she is not a good candidate for intrusive surgery. What they hope to do is a vascular radiology procedure to first hunt and find the hole, then spray something in there to seal it up.

They are envisioning weeks of antibiotics to stabilize her innards rather than days—and might even be able to send her home before they're ready. She'd have to have more of her bile going to her gut. The resistant staph draining from her side is less of a show stopper—the metabolic drain of salts might be.

However, I see this as a race between the stabilizing influence of the antibiotics and the general erosion we've seen—the leak, the growth of the abscess, and the erosion into blood vessels that are throwing blood and clots out into the drain. The leak might get much worse or I suppose the abscess could eat its way to the outside of the liver and commence leakage into her peritoneal cavity. I think the vision of the Docs here is a best-case scenario.

She has required lesser and greater amounts of oxygen, including pressurized masks, but no more respirator. Today, she's to try rice pudding and pureed foods—hope she doesn't aspirate any and kick off another round of worse pneumonia.

She's asking for visitors soon—don't see myself going for a week and a half—a lot can happen in that time frame.

◆   ◆   ◆

E-mail—Wednesday, January 2nd, 2002.
Subject: Lynda Keep Status—Day 644

The good news—Lynda is getting stable in a metabolic sense, is generally lucid, and starting tentatively back on solid foods. She is off the respirator but getting oxygen supplements. She graduated to a step-down unit.

The less good news is that her internal plumbing is still a mess, with leakage into her abscess from the bile duct and also minor blood vessels. She is losing over a liter of bile daily and these precious salts are having to be replaced by IV. She is too weak to be a good candidate for surgical correction, rather they hope to do a vascular radiology thing to hunt for the leak and spray something to seal it from the inside. This will be weeks from now rather than days, as they need these structures to stabilize under the influence of antibiotics. There is even the outside chance the antibiotics will straighten her out enough that she could go home for awhile before that procedure—in a very best of luck scenario. The question is whether with antibiotics the erosion process will halt, stabilize, or reverse.

Thanks for all the support,
-GERALD

E-mail—Friday, January 4th, 2002.
Subject: Lynda Status—Day 646.

I was surprised to learn that they tried the vascular radiology thing to plug her leak yesterday, and failed. The leak is just too big. The only options now are surgery, or going through life with a tube in her side, with a liter of bile draining daily (not a choice). I hope to hear from the actual surgeons soon as to their take on the situation, and when they'll want to try. In all other respects Lynda is stable and as strong as she's going to get, and is free of infection, so they may want to try this as early as next week.

Lynda is reportedly in good spirits, reading, and watching the snow outside her window.
-GERALD

E-mail—Friday, January 4th, 2002.
To: Liver Coordinator
Subject: Brief talk with Surgeon.

I just had an odd conversation with the Surgeon…I don't know what the working relationship your team has is, so I'll leave it in your hands as to whether there is any point to following this up any….might just be good for a laugh.

I called the Surgeon this afternoon because the Endoscopy Specialist had suggested that timing. The Surgeon told me a meeting was scheduled for Tuesday to go over the case and decide her surgical options. When I said I wanted to "be there", he at first thought I meant at the planning meeting, and when I hastened to assure him I meant "be there for the surgery" (knowing he was unaware of my geographical & domestic handicap), he obviously thought I was crazy for suggesting I might not be informed of their plans for surgery (though he handled it very diplomatically). I considered trying to explain the situation, then dropped it.

The twist I did not point out, because he obviously had nothing to do with it, is that I only found out today that Lynda had undergone the vascular procedure yesterday—and had not gone through the ritual of given consent (perhaps she did it for herself)—and had been told by the GI doctor to expect it weeks from now—and had to initiate the contact with the Endoscopy Specialist to learn of all this, this morning (following the suggestion of the nurse).

Irony abounds. Perhaps it is easier just to let the Surgeon think I'm crazy.

-GERALD

23

On Love and Obligation

	Winter	Spring	Summer	Fall
1988	(2) Engagement	(3) Wedding		
1989	(13) Reflections on Adoption			(4) Adoption
90-95	(4) Raising our Children			
1996			(5) Swelling	(1) Christmas
1997	(5) Diuretics	(5) Dehydrated	(5) Encephalopathy	(5) Encephalopathy
1998	(5) Encephalopathy	(5) Encephalopathy	(5) On the List	(6) Holding to Family
1999	(6) Holding to Family	(7) Big Crash, Shunt	(8) Dominos Falling	(9) Live Donor?
2000	(9) Aborted Hopes	(10) Transplant (11) Closing Up (12) Lingering	(13) Beacon (14) Long Distance	(14) Rehab (15) Hearing Loss (16) Home Care
2001	(16) Bile Drains	(17) Reflections—Me (18) & on the Kids (19) Insurance	(20) Abscess	(21) Finding Peace (22) Complications
2002	**(23) Love and Obligation**			

I have been called a Saint, and an Iron Man, and been told I have the strength of a Lion, for my endurance through this time of trouble. People say it is obvious that I must love Lynda very much to stay with her like this. Kind words, which stoke my pride and help lighten the burden a little bit, and true up to a point.

But I am only human and, after five years, I fear I am reaching that point, at the end of my rope, and something has changed. I'm no longer sure what to hope for. In many ways life is much easier when Lynda is away from us, and I've found to my horror that as the roller coaster goes up and down, I am greeting the "up" news with more dread than the "down". I've found that I don't want Lynda to come home, expecting that she will be a burden, though she'd be remorseful about that, expecting that she will just get sick again with the next pass of the flu bug or twist of anatomical or pharmaceutical fate, and have us all in crisis again rushing her to the hospital. It seems this will continue over and over again until she dies. It is a life I've had to endure but do not enjoy. I've run out of adrenaline and am only numb. I do not look forward to more 24/7 on-call nursing duty. If I thought Lynda might one day be healthy, I think it would be different, but now I only expect her to be pulled in and out of the hospital like she had a bunji cord attached, dragging us with her all the way, until the only peace for us all comes with her death. There was no joy left in our interactions, for me at least; Lynda still clings to the dream of returning to health and growing old with me.

Somehow I feel inside that if I really loved Lynda, I'd want her to be with us as long as possible, would endure any grief to give her a few more days or weeks with our children. I used to feel that way, and it gave me strength. I no longer feel that way, and it gives me pause. Does this mean I no longer love her?

And so I must stop and consider, what is love? What is the basis for *our* love? Yes, we had plans and agreements, but something more bound us together over the years. Is it strong enough to endure?

Let's not confuse lust with love. My back rubs *were* a strong attractor for Lynda, and we did keep each other interested at first, but that's not what brought us together; its loss can't be something that would tear us apart. Sexual activity was among the first casualties of the disease, albeit gradually; this was not something that changed recently. She has looked like a cross between my grandmother and a concentration camp survivor for a couple years now, but I've been hanging with her nonetheless; this is not new.

Nor is the explanation simple infatuation, that the young calls "love"—a crush, an obsession, a racing heart, flowers and romance. That sweetens the pot of course, and helps you hang in there in the beginning when you are full of uncertainty, but it fades quickly over the years. If the romance did not fade while keeping house together, and raising kids together, it certainly did not survive coping with the results of incontinence, the unreasonable demands born of her suffering, the waxing and waning of her spirit that left a base animal instinct in charge of her body, and then nothing. To see the object of your infatuation reduced to a poor slab of beef, all tubes, bruises, scars, and pain is not conducive to romance. Hospitals rob the patient of their dignity, and their lovers of any illusions.

Some time ago, we attended a "marriage enrichment" course through our church that stressed communication styles, but took a whack at defining love—how it is that you can be mad as hell, tired beyond thought, not even like many things about a person, and still say "I love you" and mean it. Their message was that "I love you" meant, "Despite everything else, I am still committed to you". Lynda didn't buy it. Me, I could understand how love implies commitment, but that commitment can also arise from a sense of duty, obligation, or preservation of one's self image. We all know marriages that have hung together "for the children" and indeed that had been a source of strength for me—I desperately wanted to bring my boys' mama home to them. But our wedding vows were to help each other grow and achieve, and Lynda repeatedly told me, in different ways, that I was under no obligation to stay with her—she really showed that she didn't even expect it. Friends told us that most men would not have hung around this long, and I was told repeatedly that I had exceeded everyone's expectations, that they just didn't know how I was able to hang in there. Is the national divorce rate above 50% now, even under better circumstances than we faced? I was really under no pressure from society to stay. With her own insurance and social security earnings, she wasn't even dependent on me financially.

My sense of self may have been strongest among these internal drivers. I was not one to abandon a friend in need, and I was not one to walk away from a commitment made. While others would see my weakness as "only human", it would make me feel less proud of myself. I could walk away if I knew it was the *right* thing to do. You could argue since the stress was causing me life-threateningly high blood pressure and other ill effects, and my dying would serve no good purpose, my only choice might be to distance myself in some way—at least emotionally. But this is separating the cart from the horse—my blood pressure was up, and I was stressed, precisely because I was torn by the dilemma of what to do. To plead health and walk away was to beg the question. If I did not still care about her in some way, the decision would not be hard—I would be gone, for my own health and for my own future hopes of a normal life again.

Certain writers (Heinlein first) say that love is a condition in which you care more about the well-being of another than of yourself. As an empirical observation it is true—I would not have sacrificed to the point I had if I did not love Lynda. But still, what was changing? Why were my feelings and wishes for Lynda changing in such uncomfortable ways? Was the change in me—that I had really reached a limit? Was the change in Lynda—that her illness had made her a different person, and the "real" Lynda had died with the failed surgery? Close, but it has a cheap sound of melodrama I don't like. More like, what constituted her "well being" had changed in ways that I was still grappling to understand. How could her death be viewed as a "mercy" when every fiber of her body must be fighting for survival to still be here with us, every breath she wins in the face of adversity continues to be a miracle, and in her pain and indignity she still has strength to strike out at everything around her?

I go back to that first day when Lynda was told she had a fluid mass in her abdomen, that she might have cancer. She was not afraid to die—she was afraid to abandon her children, and her first thought was of them. She wanted to leave them a purely good memory, and so we built the Train Table that first year. No, she was not afraid of death, but she was afraid of suffering. After two years of humiliation and suffering with ammonia-induced encephalopathy, her fear finally broke her, and the transplant became a symbol of salvation, rather than something to fear. This is when she realized that she might have to get very, very sick before the transplant came. This is when I lost my partner. More suffering after the transplant and she said, "If I had known what I was going to have to go through, I would never have started". Now after five years of suffering, that she would rather have died than endure, she takes refuge in her dreams, both the dream of a happy life growing old together, and the dreams she was trapped in by narcotics in the ICU. She can no longer face the burden she has been on others, no longer deal with the *pain I am in*, or to give any thought of comforting me in the ways I really need. She has slipped to a place where she can say, "I don't know why I'm still alive" (meaning both medically, and what plan God has for her). But still she fights, her body will not let go, and her dream of us together is something she grips tightly. She confusedly says she wants to come home and make life better for us, but she has no realistic plan how to do that because, realistically, she has no healthy future ahead of her. I see her hope, that can never be realized, and it rips me apart inside. She does not ask for the mercy that death would bring—why do I not hope for the impossible as she does?

The conflict is between the traumatized shell that Lynda has become and the noble person she used to be, back when she had the power to choose her own persona, her own destiny. The Lynda of five years ago would have chosen the mercy of death with dignity; the Lynda of today has been stripped of dignity and purpose. The Lynda of today simply cries out in her agony and confusion. She asks for help because death seemingly will not come.

Which Lynda do I love and hope for? They are the same, just in different circumstances. Both chose a life of dignity and purpose, though only one had it in her grasp. If "I" am a composite of my choices and values, so is she. The Lynda of today has been denied the death with dignity that the Lynda of yesterday would have chosen—all she can do is cry for help and hope to get back to the time when she was the person who was able to choose who she was. The Lynda of today only wants to be again the Lynda of yesterday—and so their wishes fall together again. The mercy of death is something the Lynda of today can no longer hope for herself directly, since it had been repeatedly denied her until now, but by hoping for it *for* her, it really is what she would want, if she again had the power of choice.

My labor of easing her suffering now simply prolongs the time that Lynda is split away from being the person she chose to be. My labor is serving no one and so has converted from a labor of love to a pointless exercise at best, a part of my loved one's torture at worst. My confusion has been over the nature of my obligation to her. To truly honor my love for her, I must choose as she does, to honor the wishes of the person she chose to be, when she had the power to do so. So I realize at last that to truly love her is to wish for the final mercy of death, knowing that to live is for her only going to be more suffering, more indignity, more thoughts of the pale shadow that she is now of the woman she once was.

What I loved about Lynda were the values *she chose* to live her life by, the courage she showed, and the impact she had on the world. These things I still love, and will remember always. Let the suffering end. Give me the strength now to continue in life in a way to make her proud of me.

24

The Final Days

	Winter	Spring	Summer	Fall
1988	(2) Engagement	(3) Wedding		
1989	(13) Reflections on Adoption			(4) Adoption
90-95	(4) Raising our Children			
1996			(5) Swelling	(1) Christmas
1997	(5) Diuretics	(5) Dehydrated	(5) Encephalopathy	(5) Encephalopathy
1998	(5) Encephalopathy	(5) Encephalopathy	(5) On the List	(6) Holding to Family
1999	(6) Holding to Family	(7) Big Crash, Shunt	(8) Dominos Falling	(9) Live Donor?
2000	(9) Aborted Hopes	(10) Transplant (11) Closing Up (12) Lingering	(13) Beacon (14) Long Distance	(14) Rehab (15) Hearing Loss (16) Home Care
2001	(16) Bile Drains	(17) Reflections—Me (18) & on the Kids (19) Insurance	(20) Abscess	(21) Finding Peace (22) Complications
2002	(23) Love, Obligation **(24) Hospice**			

Journal Entry—Sunday, January 6th, 2002

Confused and sleepy today. Allowed a "thickened liquid diet"—yogurt for instance—but not eating because she's not hungry.

◆   ◆   ◆

E-mail—Monday, January 7th, 2002
Subject: Lynda Status—Day 647

Last night there was an event which does not bode well, though it is possible there was no long-term damage. Lynda had some bleeding in the space between brain and skull, which in turn caused a seizure. She has opened her eyes a few times since, but is very much out of it, as is common for a few days after a seizure.

They have stopped the anti-coagulant and are watching to make sure she doesn't have any more bleeding. Of course the anti-coagulant was there for a reason so that's one more dimension to the balancing act.

No idea whether this sort of thing would prevent the surgery they are/were planning to discuss at a meeting tomorrow.

-GERALD

Journal Entry—Monday, January 7th, 2002

Ran over a squirrel this afternoon. My boys had school but the CNA's county shut down for snow, so I was picking up.

Talked with the Endoscopy doctor—Lynda is more alert this afternoon, recognized him, has full motor function, but is very tired. They will go ahead with discussion of her surgery, but as he put it, the question is whether the surgeons are willing to try a repair on her. He is working hard to find them an option—apparently he doesn't know yet what they *can* do for her.

◆   ◆   ◆

E-mail—Tuesday, January 8th, 2002 3:12 PM
Subject: Lynda Status—Day 648
They are going to try a radiology approach again, tomorrow or Thursday. They're going to come at the leak from the bile duct side instead of the abscess side. If this doesn't work, surgery might follow sometime next week.

-GERALD

E-mail—Wednesday, January 9th, 2002
Subject: Lynda Status—Day 649
Lynda had another seizure this morning, though CT scans show no additional bleeding. It may be a matter of regulating the anti-seizure medication better until the old blood clears out. She still has full motor function and has made short statements, but is still working back towards full alertness.

The Radiology folks are going to try once again to seal the bile duct leak TODAY.

-GERALD

Journal Entry—Thursday, January 10th, 2002

Called the Nurse this morning and she's the one who told me how things went—why didn't they call me....

◆   ◆   ◆

E-mail—Thursday, January 10th, 2002
Subject: Lynda Status—Day 650
   The attempt to repair Lynda's bile duct was aborted, as she had 2 more seizures when they tried yesterday. She had another seizure during the night and a mild one early this morning. This makes 6 altogether now. I haven't spoken to a doctor yet regarding path forward.
   Apparently the anti-seizure drugs make one lethargic, so it is futile trying to gauge her mental alertness/attention span until this all resolves.
   -GERALD

Journal Entry—Friday, January 11th, 2002

They didn't do the MRI as she had another seizure last night. They did do CT scans which showed no more bleeding!
   Now they are planning still to run the MRI...
   They are adding a second anti-seizure medication as the dilantin is apparently not getting into her at a high enough level. She apparently isn't reacting typically to the standard dose.
   She also got blood today, as her count was dropping. Why?

◆   ◆   ◆

E-mail—Monday, January 14th, 2002
Subject: Lynda Status—Day 654
   They finally got an anti-seizure medication that works for Lynda and she's been clear of them since Saturday afternoon. The MRI study showed that while her bleeding was from just one region, there were multiple spots of different age, which explains why she was having trouble for a week rather than just a few days. She is coming back out of the "dark" again, and is able to converse and interact somewhat for short periods.
   So, she's back where she was just over a week ago. They'll be trying again TODAY to do the (long-shot) vascular radiology procedure to repair her bile duct leak.

-GERALD

E-mail—Wednesday, January 16th, 2002
Subject: Lynda Status—Day 656

I'm not sure who was more confused, me or Lynda....

They have *not* yet tried to repair Lynda's bile duct leak. What was done Monday was exploratory to make sure the bile could drain somewhere if they indeed succeeded in plugging the leak. They found some defects in the ducts and so implanted a drain for her bile (to the outside). They changed out the drains again today. The actual repair attempt is in the future—any time now perhaps. Premature reports of the leak being fixed were WRONG.

As of January 8th the bugs that cultured out of her abscess were no longer staph—she had a mixture of VRE (the Vancomycin Resistant Enterocaucal bacterium that was formerly only in her gut) and something that sounds like "Stano tropa monima" so they changed around her antibiotics (she's on a mix of 3 now), and plan to test again a week from now.

They discontinued one antibiotic, "Imipentium", which could have contributed to her bleed & seizures (which have not returned since they got her on the current anti-seizure medications).

She's alert but very disoriented. Still thinks she's in Johnson City...doesn't remember anything about this hospitalization....etc. but does recognize pictures of her kids and is talking up a storm.

-GERALD

Journal Entry—Thursday, January 17th, 2002

Today I learned they are delaying the second VIR (Vascular Interventive Radiology) procedure because she is getting thick drainage from her bile duct. She may need something like Actigal to thin it or it may indicate an infection up there.

Instead they are doing an ERCP (endoscopy with anesthesia) to clean that area out and see what they find. This will be later today. The liver coordinator will be calling tomorrow with more details.

◆   ◆   ◆

Journal Entry—Friday, January 18th, 2002

Nurse says Lynda did not go to ERCP last night—they don't do those in the evening—was not scheduled—and today she is scheduled for VIR (biliary drain work) procedure. Go figure. Let's see what the coordinator comes up with.

◆   ◆   ◆

Journal Entry—Monday, January 21ˢᵗ, 2002

Got a real doctor today, and a pretty thorough review.

Lynda is alert but remains disoriented and confused (deluded was his term). There have been a lot of studies and imaging and psychiatrists and they're pretty sure it's simply the result of her experiences. They've put her back on anxiety medicine—in fact the anxiety caused at least one aborted procedure at the end of last week. They need her to chill out to work on her.

The seizures have "resolved" with addition of the second medication. He seemed to think 5-6 days rather than the nine I counted but—whatever.

The bleeding has not changed which means no new bleeds. The amount was so small there was never any "pressure" on the brain—that's good. It will take *months* to re-absorb the blood and they plan to keep her on the anti-seizure medicine for that long. They still don't know why it happened—anti-coagulants should not have caused a spontaneous bleed. But basically they're not going to worry about it *now* because there is so much else going on with her.

She had trouble with the tube feeds—nausea and vomiting and took x-rays looking for an obstruction. Today her bowel sounds are active again, swelling is down, so this seems to be resolving.

The big news is—she now has *two* abscesses! While the old one has shrunk to about 4x6 cm, this new one, formerly a "spot", is now like 3x5 cm (from the Doc's memory). Rather disturbing. While they know the bile ducts are connected to the first one, they don't know what if anything is connected to the second. They say her triple antibiotic has her covered but I'm sitting here saying—it grew with this cocktail in her veins—seems the medicine is not getting into the abscess…

In any event, these abscesses will not heal unless they can get them to drain. Recall it took months to almost resolve the first one.

They think they see "stuff" obstructing her bile duct and they need to clear that out. The Vascular Interventional Radiology (VIR) folks are going to try again tomorrow to clean it out, straighten it out, and see if they can do the sclerosis thing to plug the leak. They really do *not* want to do major surgery on her.

From my perspective, the bugs have gotten adept at hiding and eating up her liver—and there will either be nothing left of her biliary tree or there will be a "blow-out" into her abdomen eventually. They just have a very bad track record of fighting these bugs.

I still don't think she'll make it home this time but even if she does, it won't be for long.

◆   ◆   ◆

Journal Entry—Tuesday, January 22nd, 2002

They are putting her under general anesthesia with a breathing tube to try to clear out her bile duct. This will be done using the stent/drain already in place. The hope is this will help re-route the bile flow into her gut and let the leak self-repair. They will not know if this strategy is successful for a few days so the attempt to "sclerose" (scar up) her bile duct to plug the leak has been postponed until at least later in the week.

◆   ◆   ◆

E-mail—Tuesday, January 22nd, 2002
Subject: Lynda Status—Day 662

Lynda has developed a second abscess—the first has shrunk to about 4 x 6 centimeters while this new one has sprung up from a spot to now being about 3 x 5 centimeters. The old one is clearly connected to her bile duct; they don't really know much about the new one and how it is connected to whatever. They think they have a broad enough spectrum of antibiotics in her system to deal with the bugs present, and draining the abscesses is the key, but I have to note this second abscess came about while these antibiotics were in her system. I think the bugs have gotten good at hiding, and are just chewing her up.

Today they are going to try to clear some obstructions from her bile duct in hopes that they can get the bile flowing back to where it is supposed to be going, and the leak will close itself. They are going to have to put her under general anesthesia to do this, like a major surgery, though they will be working through the tubes and drains already in place. They won't know if the strategy is working for a few days so the procedure to try and plug the leak by "sclerosis" (or spraying in an agent that causes scaring to occur), second attempt, is postponed until at least the end of this week.

-GERALD

Journal Entry—Friday, January 25th, 2002

Just spoke with a psychiatrist consultant. She wanted to verify Lynda's lack of history of any mental illness. She says that "ICU psychosis" is a myth and that in

85% of the cases they found underlying medical reasons for delirium and in the remaining 15% they just think they didn't find the reason. Ergo she believes Lynda's delirium and hallucinations are a consequence of being so seriously, medically ill—directly affecting brain function—rather than being secondary. It could be any of a thousand reasons. The only cure is to resolve the medical issues.

She is eating soft foods and sleeping better.

Refused a CT scan of the head last night—very angry etc. They'll try again today.

The drain in her abscess is doing nothing—they may try to work on those or image them….?

◆   ◆   ◆

Journal Entry—Monday, January 28th, 2002

The doctor is using the term "obliterated" to describe her bile duct. Radiology has been unable to open her duct given the length of it and the way it is constricted.

Her drains are stopping up—so no telling where her bile is going. The drain in her abscess is not draining so the bugs are sitting in these untouched. She possibly won't go septic with all the antibiotics, *but*, they can't get in there and *cure* her either.

Apparently the surgeons originally said they couldn't do much to help her the first time they looked at her. The plan is to try and straighten her drains out like today and get the surgeons to reconsider her case tomorrow. These really sound like last-ditch efforts.

We're starting to talk about hospice care and putting her on just pain pills…

◆   ◆   ◆

E-mail—Monday, January 28th, 2002
Subject: Lynda Status—Day 668

We appear to be coming to the end of the road. The doctors are running out of options to keep Lynda going—her bile duct is shot, it is unclear what surgeons could do for her, and the bugs that are chewing her up from the inside out are slowly winning the battle against a raft of antibiotics.

Now, Lynda is protesting against anything further being done to her. She just wants the suffering to stop.

I am going down tomorrow, Tuesday, to consult first hand and see what our path forward from here is. I don't expect to be at work the next couple weeks. My cell phone is probably the best way to get a message to me—I'll be booking a room at the usual hotel near the transplant center.

  -GERALD

Journal Entry—Tuesday, January 29th, 2002

Packing up to go to the transplant center this morning with my older boy. The CNA is going to make the round trip Wednesday and bring him home. My folks are flying out Thursday. It all seems unreal. I guess that's why we're going—to make it seem more real and unavoidable.

Evening—The doctor confirmed all my suppositions—plus added a couple of logs to the fire. Her right portal vein is clotted off again. While this does not stop nourishment of that part of the liver, it probably does restrict flow of antibiotic to that region, and affects the growth of the abscesses. They can't use anticoagulants to battle this, because of the brain bleeds. The other thing is her urine has in it strains of multi-resistant bacteria so it is spreading.

Lynda very quickly accepted that "no bile duct" meant she was going to die. She seems split between two points of view—one that if she is going to die anyway, there was no point to the tests and procedures, so she gleefully waved them all off. On the other hand she felt "unprepared" and wanted 2-3 days to say goodbye to everybody.

She was quite alert and processing well—clear speech. But, she had a hard time with context and would misread words into her own context—"drink" instead of "drain" and go off on a tangent. She also would hear things and think someone is in the room and start talking to them. She thought our younger son, her own mom, and several other people were in the room while we were there.

Even Later—Lynda was much harder to communicate with. The male nurse offered her a TV dinner and somehow she concluded that he made them himself. So she got off on all these business ventures and recipes he could use—largely because she was still totally convinced I had lost my job. I couldn't get her to change the subject. I think food was so dominant in her thinking because she had been mostly NPO since the previous day for the drain-changing procedure which kept getting postponed. So she could eat again up until midnight, and she did—lots—and well. I don't know what the lack of bile is going to do to her but she had steak tips in gravy.

She seemed totally oblivious to our previous discussions about her fate, and kept talking to our youngest son who was not actually there. Finally as we were leaving to put the *boys* (allegedly plural) to bed, she said "We'll deal with all this together because we're still a family—*at least for a few more days*!!" So she is aware of her situation and accepting it.

◆   ◆   ◆

Journal Entry—Wednesday Night, January 30th, 2002

She pulled out her bile duct drain and Foley catheter and would have pulled out her central IV line (and bled to death) if they hadn't restrained her and given her *two* doses of Haldol.

She is clearly saying, "Enough!"

She slept off most of Thursday and had very calm discussions Thursday night with Auntie, then with all of us Friday, making funeral arrangements etc. We've pretty much got all the details worked out.

Her brother came in Friday night—the last of the visitors.

◆   ◆   ◆

Journal Entry—Saturday, February 2nd, 2002

They're going to stop the antibiotics today. She's starting to get itchy again from bile build-up. Going septic would be a much more peaceful way to go. We'll do everything we can to make her comfortable. Who knows, maybe the morphine pump arrangement will lead to an overdose again—which would be even better.

◆   ◆   ◆

E-mail—Monday, February 4th, 2002
Subject: Lynda Status—Day 675—2 days off antibiotics.

Got quick access to e-mail. Darn I hate being right, but I'm sorry to confirm my e-mail of last week—this is the end of the road for Lynda.

Lynda's bile duct is not just leaking, it is scarred too much to reopen. There are no surgical options that make sense. They were trying to buy her time with a drain to take off the bile but in an act of saying "Enough!", Lynda ripped the drain out Wednesday night. They had to restrain and sedate her to prevent her pulling out her central IV line.

She was lucid for several out-of-town visitors up through the weekend, and remains fairly so today but, as the bile builds up in her system, she is starting to get jaundiced and itch like crazy. Also she's developing back pain from the internal pressures.

They stopped the antibiotics on Saturday and all that remains is to keep her as comfortable as possible with anti-itch and painkillers, and hope that peace comes soon.

My folks are with the boys back home so everything is under control there.

Pray for us—but pray for peace.

-GERALD

After making an important decision like stopping Lynda's antibiotics, it is natural to expect something dramatic to happen. Of course antibiotics take time to clear out of the body, and once gone, merely stop being a check on some other process that takes time to establish itself. As was my tendency, I tried to get a handle on this uncertainty in order to best prepare myself emotionally for the most likely possibilities.

On the pessimistic side, I had seen Lynda go from apparently doing great to being in a hospital setting with doctors doing intensive things to her on numerous occasions. If this was any guide, it would take at least 3 days for Lynda to die, 4 if you allow a day for the antibiotics to clear. In this scenario, why upset her and make her uncomfortable by moving her around and uprooting her familiar setting.

On the optimistic side, I had to hearken back to the events around Thanksgiving for a reference. Then, the doctors thought her abscess was almost gone and thus thought it safe to stop her antibiotics, which they had to do for the clot problem. It was 19 days from such a clean start that she went jaundiced etc. So I figured the upper limit was 3 weeks; Lynda was *not* starting from a clean cold start here. Three weeks though was a long time, and perhaps different arrangements were in order.

Three days or three weeks—what a difference. I had headed to the Transplant Center thinking that if we had to take that step, of turning off the antibiotics, then I would definitely be a week right there at the hospital. If things progressed such that I would have to be longer, then I'd work it out from there.

Lynda really wanted to go home to die in her own bed, in comfortable and familiar surroundings. I could understand the desire to get away from the hospital, but I don't think she understood what she was asking in terms of the consequences on others.

She had told me stories about her sitting with infants when they turned off life support in the neonatal intensive care units. She would sit and wait with them, and the parents, for the end. This was obviously an important thing for her and I was prepared to be there in the hospital to perform that one last duty for her. I was less well prepared to sit by her bedside at home and nurse her for 3 weeks with only intermittent visits from a visiting nurse—but I guess I could have done that if necessary.

What I balked at was the idea of her doing that in our house with the children there. My youngest was already getting scared and clingy, wouldn't go downstairs alone, and was already jumping and startling when he lost track of who was where in the house. Can you imagine what it would be like for him to live in the house *where his mother had died?* I don't think I could let that happen and I don't think she was thinking about the impact on her boys when she made that request. I had to be strong and resist and explain.

After the first handful of days, where Lynda was strong and showing no signs of infection—or even bad jaundice really—the question came to the front. I was prepared to sit with her there in the hospital a while longer, but the doctors were clearly unhappy with that plan. They just didn't see her as dying real soon, and were concerned that this was not the best setting for making the best of her last days. They had some specific suggestions that hit home—hospice programs were better at grief and pain management, and had programs that offered, as a part of the paid package, counseling services for the rest of the family for 12-18 months afterward. We would not get those benefits if Lynda died in the hospital.

I knew nothing about the Hospice movement at that point in my life. Hospice was a movement that focused on treating the symptoms of discomfort, thus letting patients have a more dignified and meaningful end to their lives.

Ultimately we came to view hospice as a good compromise, closer to home with flexibility to come and go, closer to the larger body of visitors Lynda would get back home, but not so intrusive with the grosser medical aspects into the boys' last sanctuary.

E-mail—Tuesday, February 5th, 2002
Subject: Lynda Status—Day 676—3 days off antibiotics
The doctors think Lynda may last another week or two (or more) so we are transferring to the Hospice House near home—this evening.

I don't know any more details but visitors will be very welcome.

Lynda is having a hard time reading and "Backgammon" was outrageous, but she is still pretty clear, and herself. The itches and pains are still under control of medications.
-GERALD

E-mail—Sunday, February 10th, 2002
Subject: Lynda Status—Day 681—8 days off antibiotics.

Lynda is feeling well with the change in surroundings and the absence of immune suppressants and antibiotics in her system (temporary relief of course). She has been out to eat, to synagogue, touring the nearby downtown historic district by wheelchair and hopes to take her boys to the go-kart place this afternoon!!!

Her VCO (voice carry over, with a translator in the loop to type your words) phone is installed and working so if you want to try long distance contact, I recommend calling the nurse's station and asking Lynda to call OUT on the VCO.

Lynda seems comfortable and at peace for her final days. Always unfinished business, particularly her boys, but such is life for everyone, if we only knew.

Take care, all!
-GERALD

Hospice turned out to be a marvelous place—not just the facilities but the people. The people who work in hospice have a very special understanding of the meaning of life, and help their patients to find that as well towards the end. All seem to be very religious, but never sought to impose their views; they were happy to see Lynda actively practicing her Jewish traditions, saying they were just glad that she had a faith to find comfort in. They were very helpful and accommodating—and all got a special thrill out of Lynda because they never got to see patients so full of energy and life as Lynda. She was the first to ever use their huge Jacuzzi tub and everyone had a blast when they put in too much bubble bath. A tremendous stream of people came to visit Lynda—when she was not out gadding about the countryside. Lynda turned the nurses into her personal social secretaries to keep her busy schedule, and they were happy to do it. All in all it was a strangely happy time, for all the grim thoughts and preparations—for it was also "a house of tears." I can't thank the hospice workers enough—in fact Lynda penned a thank-you to them that she wanted us to print in the newspaper posthumously.

Eventually everyone said their goodbyes and the stream turned into a trickle. A small but dedicated core group helped me by staying the night with Lynda in turns so that between us we never left her alone a single night. Lynda insisted that she would be fine with the wonderful nurses, but I'm sure she appreciated having old friends with her.

And still she hung on. I read a book called "Final Gifts" which speaks of the dying and how they tend to cling to life until some last unresolved issue is dealt with so that they can pass peacefully. But identifying the issues is not easy and what we, the survivors, need to do is listen for the clues that tell us where the rub is, to help our loved ones find a final peace.

Ultimately Lynda's final peace seemed to focus on spending her last birthday at our time-share in Williamsburg.

E-mail—Tuesday, February 12th, 2002
Subject: Lynda Status—Day 683—10 days off antibiotics.

Lynda is starting to get a bit more confused, so the bugs may be getting a firmer hold. With the confusion comes some depression—she's wanting to avoid a lot of visitors at this point—says it makes her sad—trying to go out as much as possible—so do call ahead before dropping in. Things might be changing rapidly from here forward.

-GERALD

Journal Entry—Friday, February 15th, 2002 —13 days off antibiotics.

What a strange and wonderful time this has been. Without the secondary effects of the antibiotics and immune suppressants dragging her down, Lynda has been alert, lively, and free of pain, hallucinations, and delusions. She has had a stream of nearly a dozen visitors daily, and gotten out for many restaurant meals—and cooked macaroni and cheese for the boys. Other activities range from taking the boys Go-Kart racing to visiting synagogue. I had her out in the downtown historic district in a wheelchair to tour, but she's walking pretty well and going full speed ahead.

We see little signs and hints of increasing confusion but not enough that a stranger would notice. Her jaundice is not severe—possibly due to the effects of the anti-itch medications.

However, without the antibiotics it's just a matter of time before she goes septic.

The Hospice House has been great—the place and the people. We couldn't imagine a better setting if you've got to walk this walk.

◆   ◆   ◆

E-mail—Friday, February 15, 2002

To: Lynda's Brother

The Docs recommended hospice because they thought it would be weeks, rather than days, before she went septic. She is showing increased signs of confusion, lost words, slower speech, etc. but is going great guns still. Plans to make it to synagogue tonight.

She is puffing up fluid-wise because of her lack of an outlet for the bile, but is not really in pain (is taking no pain killers) and the itching is controlled well via medication.

To look at how "alive" she is without the side effects of the antibiotics and immune suppressants in her system, you'd think she was doing great, or had rallied somehow, but really without them it is just a matter of time.

E-mail—Monday, March 4th, 2002
Subject: Lynda Status—Day 703

Four weeks off antibiotics now, Lynda is continuing to surprise us by hanging on and gripping life with both hands. In some ways she is reconciled to her medical situation, and is viewing this time as a gift to use for tidying up her unfinished business and saying her goodbyes. On the other hand, she says she'll go down fighting—that's just her.

The long-range prognosis is unchanged. We don't know whether the bugs will get her by making her go septic, by causing liver failure, or by causing fluid buildup that presses on her heart and lungs. They say she could remain stable for totally unpredictable amounts of time, then take some sudden and irreversible drops for the worse to lower plateaus and re-stabilize…

Right now, Lynda has very slightly slurred speech and tires very, very easily—but she's still herself. Her appetite is extraordinary. I did not want to push anybody away that feels the need to visit. Be forewarned—she tries to get out every day for anything from lunch, playing with the boys, shopping, cooking supper at the house, anything and everything so *call ahead, as there is a real risk of her not being there*! She has even set herself the goal of going to Williamsburg this year for her birthday in 3-4 weeks, and I'm told this can be arranged if she is still on this same "plateau" and physically able to do it.

Phoning instructions for the VCO and directions to hospice attached—
-GERALD

Journal Entry—Thursday, March 7, 2002

Coming up on five weeks now without antibiotics and I'm exhausted. Lynda is not showing much of any jaundice—very gray in fact. She has fluid and swelling problems, but the worst is her mental confusion. She's still herself and puts on a good front, but challenging mental tasks are getting harder and harder. We're playing a lot of Backgammon and it's a good indicator of her mental status. She cheats outrageously and doesn't even realize it; she thinks she's getting better and better but really she's moving twice, counting repeatedly until it comes out the way she wants, moves the first die then the second then the first again, moves 4 *pairs* of numbers when she gets doubles and so forth.

She has gotten bad enough to be difficult to manage. She has these grandiose plans that then fail in her attempt to execute. She bought a fondue pot for $3 at a garage sale then tried to make it without a recipe—what a disaster! Then a couple days later she threw out the fondue pot along with our older boy's camping Sterno, scout membership card, and my mail stack, etc.

Also she's lost the ability to show consideration for others easily—she just doesn't realize how much trouble she's putting us through or how awkward she makes it.

Now today the Doctor hinted that he wants to do CT scans to see what's really going on inside—the bile is obviously draining. "Hand of God," he says.

So now maybe she'll be living quite a while? This is going to kill *me*! I just can't take this continuing level of emotional intensity.

I spent much of the day at work figuring out if I could quit my day job to get away from the stress—and just write and care for the boys. The answer is I could actually, if I sell the house and move into something half the value (inside city limits for school bus). Then the boys' college is paid for and with social security and interest off investments (including life insurance from Lynda), I could make ends meet. One car. Pay for Blue Cross under the COBRA laws ($700/month). The catch is we couldn't afford the CNA at all, and the boys have become really attached to her. I guess I feel like I need some *reason* to put up with the stress, and I'm not finding it easily. I really need to take care of myself and that might just mean collapsing into my emotional shell and not coming out for a long while. Not good for the boys, but it is an emotional balm to know that I *could*. It wouldn't do them any good if I blew a gasket either—my blood pressure has been as high as 150/105 when I wake up in the morning.

Then up pops the idea that Lynda may linger on a *lot* longer, with her not-so-bad state—no way to escape work, no way to escape the stress. I suppose that should be good news, but I can't keep riding this roller coaster.

…Five weeks now off antibiotics; she had exceeded my most optimistic esti-mates and physically looked great—mobile, not yellow, and full of energy. She needed few pain pills. Only the vague specter of slipping mental function, which she concealed well, indicated an ongoing problem, and that was rather subjective. We all began to doubt her condition was really terminal, and maybe a miracle was happening. To deal with it day by day, I had to keep repeating to myself that she was only this good because she was off the antibiotics; she was living on borrowed time. It got me through the days, but there was always a little voice of self-doubt. Thus the ground was laid for more emotional bricks I would have to deal with later.

◆   ◆   ◆

Letter to Lynda—Friday, March 8th, 2002

Lynda,

I'd like to update you on some discussion I've had with the hospice doctor and the liver coordinator (who talked with the liver doctors).

The hospice doctor is puzzled at how well you are doing, and was suggesting tests (CT scan) to learn more about what's going on inside you. The transplant center doctors have said it would be academic and that the results would not affect the course of your situation or your treatment.

Some points:

- Your bile must *mostly* be draining through the bad bile duct, as you are not all *that* yellow, your blood work is not all *that* bad, and your stools are brown.

- The hospice doctor wondered if your abscesses might be gone, but the transplant doctors don't think that is at all possible. Personally, watching your mental alertness progression over time, I think the toxins are building up slowly.

- The hospice doctor apparently doesn't think you need to be at hospice house at this time. You are *not* going to a nursing home—but they might want to push for you to leave the hospice house setting. The best option seems to be to send you home for awhile, and then move back to hospice when it becomes more appropriate later.

- While I am concerned about you dying right there in front of the boys, I agree that things will move slowly enough that we can manage that issue at home.

- We need to work a bit on arrangements—I don't want to lose the social worker's services for the boys, for instance.

- The liver coordinator is canceling your March 18th annual follow-up appointments at the transplant center. If your immune system by some miracle fights the bugs into a stalemate situation for some number of months, we might have to start doing blood work to determine need for Prograf again.

You seem to be granted the gift of more time than we had hoped was possible. I'm glad you're able to make the most of it.

Love always,
    -GERALD

Journal Entry—Midnight, March 9-10, 2002

Coming home from wrestling match 2 hours from home...

I'm physically and emotionally exhausted—kind of at the end of my rope. I was adjusting to the idea of Lynda coming home for awhile per the hospice doctor, but his timing really stinks.

Now, as I tried to explain the situation to Lynda, she has gone into that hateful stage where nothing works and everybody else gets blamed for it. I'm supposedly a horrible monster for asking her to slow down and not burden me (by not volunteering to cater any *more* Friday night banquets). I'm accused of wanting her to die so I can go find some other woman to be with. The worst of it is there is some truth to it—I do want it to be over—I can't take it any more. But finding another woman? A month ago that was an appealing challenge but now I've been ground down so much all I want to do is crawl into my shell and lick my wounds. My future looks pretty bleak and lonely as I don't see myself exposing my tender wounded psyche to the emotional bumper cars of trying to get to know a hundred women and sort through which *one* of them might be a good mate for me. I don't feel like I could take that kind of risk.

All I can do is hang on, try to ignore Lynda's grosser moments, and pretend it isn't happening as it eats me up. I feel like the little Spartan boy hiding a fox beneath his tunic.

◆   ◆   ◆

Note to CNA and Hospice Staff—March 18th, 2002

Since Lynda spoke of draining fluid to you then spoke of hoping for a miracle to change her prognosis to me, I tried to discuss these issues with her.

She was pretty obtuse about recognizing what I meant in terms of a "deep" discussion.

When I specified discussing her medical condition, she said she didn't want to talk about possibilities in advance; she'd deal with it when it really came up.

When I pointed out the line of her questions, and asked if she wanted to talk about buying time with medical intervention, needles, etc. she said, "It's a terrible thing watching your faculties go."

This tells me she does *not* want to do anything to prolong the process of watching her faculties degrade—*and* that she's aware of what's happening to her.

Thought you'd like to know...

-GERALD

E-mail—Friday, March 22nd, 2002
Subject: Lynda Status—Day 721—7 weeks off antibiotics.

Well, Lynda is still hanging on. Despite some worrying signs to those who know her best, she insists she feels fine and certainly doesn't need skilled nursing care on a 24/7 basis. This latter is also the opinion of the insurance companies (I'm not sure they know she had her hair done yesterday, but certainly are aware of her daily outings). Bottom line is, until she really DOES need that level of care...

LYNDA IS MOVING BACK HOME TODAY! She'll have a week to rest up, then, Lord willing, we're doing the Williamsburg thing.

You just never know. Every day is a gift....

-GERALD

◆　　　◆　　　◆

Journal Entry—Wednesday, March 27th, 2002

A couple nights ago Lynda made macaroni and cheese from scratch. Lynda told our oldest boy that she'd be happy to teach him how to make it so that he'd always know that there would be something he could make to eat. She's trying to take care of him after she's gone—trying to be sure he never starves!

The CNA says that Lynda's been laughing more the last couple days than any time she has ever known Lynda.

◆　　　◆　　　◆

It had been an amazing and completely unforeseen eight weeks off antibiotics. Lynda was full of life and energy. It appeared that she would get her wish of celebrating one last birthday with the family at Williamsburg. We had surprised her the first year we had the timeshare by decorating the place with balloons and crepe paper, and made a big to-do with an ice cream cake and presents we had bought in the Colonial ships. It became an annual tradition, which I'm sure we'll observe in some form every year that we go.

◆　　　◆　　　◆

Journal Entry—Thursday, March 28th, 2002

Day before we are to leave for Williamsburg, of course is when it hits. Lynda is spiking a fever of 102 (Tylenol brings down to 101.5). If it is a blocked bile duct that clears itself again, she and I might follow the crew shortly. If it is permanently blocked or bacterial sepsis coming, it's the beginning of the end.

◆　　　◆　　　◆

Journal Entry—Saturday, March 30th, 2002

Well, we seem to have crossed a new threshold today. It's 5:00 pm and Lynda has not woken up at all. No medicines, no fluids, no opening of eyes. I don't think she'll be able to cross back from this. I've tried several times to rouse her gently but there is almost no response. She seems a bit easier when I stroke her hair, but then she's not uncomfortable.

She takes one big deep breath every 5 seconds or so, then lets it out with a loud sigh. Sometimes she rattles a little on fluid or a snore.

I don't think she was up at all during the night so I think we're looking at 18 hours asleep now.

This morning she felt cool, now she feels warmer as if a fever is building up again.

This all started Thursday. She woke up somewhat glassy-eyed and shortly after lunch spiked a fever of over 102 (where she normally runs 96-97). Her words were more tangled and she was quite upset at the notion that she might miss Williamsburg. She was so very tired she kept falling asleep (literally falling off the chair) while they were painting her nails—red and white stripes with a blue field with stars.

She tried to show our oldest boy what she had had done to her nails and in her tongue-tied state called it "Williamshand".

Friday her fever was mostly controlled by Tylenol, though she still appeared yellow and she had head-aches which required Roxanol to control. She slept most of the day but was most alert when my brother with his new wife and two step-children showed up. We packed my boys and my Mom up for the seven of them to go on to Williamsburg.

We left it that "maybe" we could follow the next day if her fever stayed down—there seemed a chance this could have been caused by a temporarily blocked bile duct that had again cleared.

The minute they left, she had us run down the hill for chicken carry-out and a couple movies. (She had been insisting that she was going to cook this big batch of chicken for us, so had chicken on the mind).

She couldn't stay awake through the first movie and asked me to help her to bed. That might have been around 7:00pm. I got her evening pills about 10:00pm or so—she'd been dozing and reading. That's the last she was awake to my knowledge.

I slept quite soundly so if she got up in the night, bad balance and all, I wasn't awake or aware enough to know.

This timing is probably for the best, as the CNA points out. This way Lynda gets to die at home as she wanted, and the kids aren't here to deal with it.

Tomorrow is the 2nd anniversary of her transplant, though I don't think that has a lot of significance to her.

You'd like to think this timing was chosen to spare the boys but right up to the last minute she clung to her hope of getting to Williamsburg for her birthday. The last words of significance I can recall from last night were, "Are you still okay for Williamsburg tomorrow?" or something to that effect.

I think the stress of the build-up may have finally gotten to her. I don't think she achieved her final goal that she had set for herself and was bitterly disappointed. She had spoken of how the last five years had been "wait and see," and she was upset by that.

Come 6:00pm I'll start spreading the word of her condition.

◆   ◆   ◆

E-mail—Saturday, March 30th, 2002
Subject: Lynda Status—Day 729

Well, Lynda seems to have crossed a threshold today, 1 day shy of the 2nd anniversary of her transplant. Basically, she hasn't woken up today at all—that's 18 hours of sleep as of this writing. She is breathing deeply and seems comfortable, but of course is not taking fluids or medication.

Gentle attempts to rouse her are unsuccessful. I don't think she'll be crossing back from this one, as much as she fought to go to Williamsburg for her Birthday. The last thing of any significance she said was to ask if I was still okay with us leaving for Williamsburg this next morning.

The boys went ahead to Williamsburg with Grandma and my brother, so they are in good hands. I'll try to send out word when the end arrives, but it won't be much longer now.

Thanks for all the support.

-GERALD

Saturday evening I called the hospice nurse. Lynda had been asleep for 24 hours. Of course they came right out to see for themselves.

Lynda had spent the entire day in the same identical position—along the right edge of the bed, limbs straight down, with her head turned to the right. The main thing the nurse really wanted to do was shift her onto her left side so that she wouldn't be as likely to aspirated her fluids, and also put a pad under her. She wanted to put in a catheter as well, but didn't have one with her.

Lynda protested in her sleep over being moved, but seemed to settle down before the nurse left. But, that had broken her out of her sleep. Not long after the nurse left, Lynda called out and I came to find her trying to sit up in bed. She was shaking like a leaf—actually in big rolling waves like she had no control over her body. She said, "Help me!" and fixed her attention on the bathroom door. So, I tried to help her stand up, but her legs buckled. Eventually I just picked her up bodily and put her back on the bed, mildly straining my back. Then I just sat there and calmed her down by stroking her hair, feeling terrible that I couldn't help her, and in fact was waiting, doing nothing to stop it, while she died. About the point when she calmed down, the nurse returned with a catheter. After hearing my story, though, she decided to leave well enough alone.

Two hospice nurses came out the next morning, Easter Sunday, and gave her a bath with no response from her at all, unlike the night before.

Auntie was able to come before the end. She had been planning to drive to meet us in Williamsburg so could easily reroute to our home instead. All day Sunday Lynda rattled and gurgled as she labored with her breathing. That evening we heard a change in her breathing, perhaps less labored, and went in to check on her together. We watched as she took her last breath and simply remained peacefully still. We waited five minutes, and then called the nurses back. Lynda had finally passed away. It was not the shock one might expect, but rather we tiptoed around, with a sense of disbelief. Lynda was finally gone.

E-mail—Monday, April 1st, 2002

Subject: Lynda—Final Day

Lynda passed away peacefully last evening at 9:25 pm. Two sleep-filled days after she succumbed to the effects of the bacteria in her system, she simply stopped breathing. This was the second anniversary of her transplant.

The funeral will be sometime Tuesday, mid-day or afternoon followed by a burial service.

NO FLOWERS PLEASE. In lieu of flowers, a memorial fund for "programs for children" has been established called the "Lynda Pearl Keep Early Intervention Memorial". Donations can be made via "ETSU Foundation, Box 70721, Johnson City, TN 37614".

-GERALD

We had a fine funeral in which Lynda's accomplishments and her character as a person were honored and cherished. Lynda had touched many lives, from infants to adults. We will all miss her very much but she'll never be completely gone. The ripples she caused will spread out and live on in all of us.

25

Grief

	Winter	Spring	Summer	Fall
1988	(2) Engagement	(3) Wedding		
1989	(13) Reflections on Adoption			(4) Adoption
90-95	(4) Raising our Children			
1996			(5) Swelling	(1) Christmas
1997	(5) Diuretics	(5) Dehydrated	(5) Encephalopathy	(5) Encephalopathy
1998	(5) Encephalopathy	(5) Encephalopathy	(5) On the List	(6) Holding to Family
1999	(6) Holding to Family	(7) Big Crash, Shunt	(8) Dominos Falling	(9) Live Donor?
2000	(9) Aborted Hopes	(10) Transplant (11) Closing Up (12) Lingering	(13) Beacon (14) Long Distance	(14) Rehab (15) Hearing Loss (16) Home Care
2001	(16) Bile Drains	(17) Reflections—Me (18) & on the Kids (19) Insurance	(20) Abscess	(21) Finding Peace (22) Complications
2002	(23) Love, Obligation (24) Hospice	(25) Grieving		

I had an enlightening experience today in church.

It had been a month since Lynda's funeral, and life had settled back into a routine. Attending church again, for the third time, seeing old familiar faces, was just part of the process of seeking out community again after the long isolation; it was an obvious thing I knew I must do, and so had started in a tentative way. The boys were still somewhat listless, not eating well, and not sleeping well, but they were talking about their mother so the healing process was proceeding. I had the same symptoms, though I was less sure what healing I was going to need. Only three times in 30 days had I relived, through a dream, the nightmare of watching Lynda's final gut-wrenching slide to the end—the final disintegration of her as a person as her mind went. I could guess at what psychological traumas might manifest in me, but I could not yet see it clearly. I was too busy, too numb.

I had been lead to expect a sharp shock with the actual final passing of Lynda, but this did not occur. I rationalize that having grieved for her so many times before, I was more apt to wonder if it was real this time, rather than be surprised. My most intense break-down level of emotions came not when thinking about Lynda, or even my own future challenges of coping with her loss, but when thinking of the boys. Lynda accomplished much in life, and made every minute count. While her ending was sad, and the path she took was hard to contemplate, her plight was no longer emotionally overwhelming me. For myself, I was a big boy and would cope—I had a measure of freedom that married men sometimes envy in bachelors, and at worst I was depressed by the long hard road I might face to finding a true partner again. The thought that the boys were without a mother still made my heart rise to my throat, but I had been dealing with that thought for a year and a half and I think I understood it, had done what I could about my feeling, and for the boys, putting in place the best support network I could. I had secured the closest proximity of potential mother-surrogates that I could manage. I thought I had that as well under control as anyone could expect me to have done. I had written 130 thank-you notes to the attendees of the funeral and could express myself coolly when speaking of Lynda's passing.

So there I was in church, thinking I had attained a level of equilibrium. I knew that out there on the horizon—the three-month point they say—I would be facing a time of extreme loneliness, after the deluge of sympathetic offerings had abated. I had said all along, not quite in jest, that I was the sort to be rock-steady in the crunch, then fall apart later. This was clearly true in each short episode we had faced. I was waiting for the big crash at the end now, and didn't know whether I had over-rated my likely reaction, or I had a dark period of morose hermitage ahead of me, where I collapsed in on myself socially, and licked my wounds—or worse. I seemed not to be dealing with anything pressing at the moment, and was dutifully partaking of outside company to ease the hurt.

Our church services have a segment called "candles of community" where anyone taken by the spirit can light a candle and share a joy or concern with the rest of the congregation. It was my third time back, and I figured I was ready to light a candle for Lynda; I only had to decide what I was going to say to the congregation.

There was one seemingly minor thing that was troubling me, which I could throw out for community scrutiny—perhaps drawing back some advice. This was the matter of setting a headstone on Lynda's grave. I was surprised, having gone through the funeral arrangements, to realize that no one had broached the issue of a headstone in making arrangements. I felt this was an oversight, and felt the desire and duty to immediately pursue an appropriate headstone. Also, a friend of mine whose opinion mattered much to me, had expressed a poor opinion of an acquaintance who had completely neglected to place headstones for a wife and child he had buried. But on the other hand, this same friend told me that Lynda had wanted the first anniversary of her death to be marked by the placing of a headstone; this was news to me. Lynda had asked for a traditional Jewish service, but had interpreted things in her own fashion as well. Working with the synagogue's cemetery committee, I learned that indeed they "recommended" a wait of at least nine months. I had asked the rabbi about why this was custom, and he told me that eleven months fit with the schedule of the ritual mourning period that Jews traditionally followed in sitting "Shiva". This struck the best balance of grieving for and remembering the departed one. I was uncomfortable with leaving Lynda without a headstone for so long; it seemed to me that I was neglecting a duty. But on the other hand, she had requested the delay.

So it was that I thought to lay the tension of this decision on the laps of the congregation as a way they could share in my feelings of sorrow and concern, the tension over deciding the best way to balance grieving over and honoring Lynda. I clearly wanted to do it sooner, and thought to "justify" this somehow by pointing to how long I had already been grieving for Lynda over the up and down course of her illness—that this time somehow ought to "count" towards the requisite eleven months, somehow. It had been one month since Lynda had passed away. It had been 3 months since we gave up on her and stopped the antibiotics, moving to a hospice program. It had been 4 months since I had considered an experimental surgery to be a legitimate way for Lynda to escape the suffering. If you add up the segments of time over the illness when I had no hope, it ran to well over half a year. The first time I had given up hope of her making it home was almost 2 years ago. I had lost her as a supportive partner when she was consumed by the terror over 3 years ago. The first time we had faced the possibility of her dying was five and a half years ago. Hadn't I spent enough time grieving for Lynda already? This was the first time I had let my heart, rather than my head, feel the weight of the burden I had been carrying this whole long horrible and lonely time. My eyes watered over and I could not face the congregation. I could not even stand up and light a candle for Lynda, even saying only that it had been a month, or even say nothing. I cried most of the rest of the service, a slow weepy cry. Even as I write this, four hours later, after thinking about how I would describe my feelings on paper, I feel the overwhelming sense of my heart rising in my chest, my lips getting thick, and my eyes shutting down on me. I now feel the wound that my mind said must be there. I now know that I am a crushed and battered remnant of the strong person I've tried to be all these years.

What have I got to show for this terrible sacrifice? Lynda is gone. Perhaps I set an example for the boys, though I now feel overwhelmed by the responsibility I have to them. The most I can do for them now is to help steady them, as they prepare to fly from the nest. I can be proud of what I have done, and draw strength from that, but the hurt diminishes me more, at least for now. Others were watching and may understand me to one degree or another, but everyone has troubles of their own to deal with. Perhaps my experience will help others face their own challenges with greater courage, and hence I may become their hero. But who can see both my worth and my need, and still be free enough of their own troubles to help me with mine? Who can understand and care for me now? I feel very alone. Lynda left many positive things behind, but she also left a hole in my heart and my life.

The hardest measure of my courage will be how I face the challenge of healing and going on. Will it be alone, or will I have the courage to risk more hurt by seeking help, finding new strength in human companionship? Only time will tell.

978-0-595-36814-3
0-595-36814-X

www.ingramcontent.com/pod-product-compliance
Lightning Source LLC
Chambersburg PA
CBHW030308290526
45785CB00001B/261

* 9 7 8 0 5 9 5 3 6 8 1 4 3 *